Little to Say – Much to Tell

Little to Say – Much to Tell

Speech, Language and Hearing Problems in Books, Films and Theater

---

Eric Manders

Eric Manders

Little to Say – Much to Tell.

Speech, Language and Hearing Problems in Books, Films and Theater

ISBN 13: 979-8-5367-2058-5

Imprint: Independently published

Contents

Introduction

Through the years thousands of books have been written and hundreds of films have been made in which all kinds of diseases, disorders and impairments play an important role. This shouldn't be surprising since medical problems have a major impact on our daily functioning and on a person's quality of life. Usually the term health related quality of life (HRQoL) is used in this context. In line with this, speech, language and hearing disorders have also often been the subject of books, theater performances and films.

In this book we will give a description of what has appeared on this subject in the so-called popular media. In addition to providing an overview and a description, we also tried to include some critical comments where appropriate. Another aim is to examine how persons with different kinds of communication disorders are described and perceived in films, books and other media.

It was not our aim to be complete. The amount of published material is simply too large for that, which means we were forced to make a selection. We drew some inspiration from the book '*Dysfluencies: on speech disorders in modern literature*' (Eagle, 2014), which is, to our knowledge, one of the only publications on this subject in the last decade. We also found a lot of information on the internet (a selected list of websites we consulted can be found as an appendix), including a lot of summaries and reviews of books and trailers of films we have discussed. It is easy to understand it would have been practically impossible to read all the books described and to watch all the movies discussed.

The title '*Little to say, much to tell*' wasn't chosen just like that. First of all a lot of characters described in books or presented in films have difficulty speaking, causing them to speak very little or even not at all. However many of them have much to tell, even if they have to use means other than spoken language!

As we will see, in popular media people with speech, language and hearing problems are often portrayed negatively and pejoratively. They are also frequently and incorrectly considered as inferior. We found that the opposite is often true: many of them are brilliant and very smart individuals.

We made a classification based on the different conditions and problems described. The first three chapters will focus on aphasia, locked-in syndrome and dysarthria. These can be considered as neurogenic communication disorders. Chapter four and five deal with stuttering and mutism respectively, being rather psychogenic problems, albeit not always. Hearing loss and deafness are the subject of chapter six. In the final chapter some other communication disorders such as cleft palate, voice problems, articulation and child language disorders will be discussed. We have always made a distinction between (auto)biographic and non-fiction books and films on the one hand and fictional stories and films on the other. Where appropriate we also included children's books and young adult fiction.

We deliberately did not focus on specialized professional publications, as we are convinced that specialists in the respective fields know perfectly where to find those. Nor did we choose to include speech and language disorders, which are the result of broader, primary problems such as dementia, autism or intellectual disabilities. Although we realize that these also give cause for communication problems, we have decided to leave them outside the scope of this book. An awful lot of books and films are made about autism, and the same goes for dementia. It would have led us too far to describe all of these.

We would like to express our gratitude to everyone who gave us valuable tips during our search and who helped us complete this publication.

Chapter 1: Aphasia

Aphasia can be defined as an acquired language disorder, caused by brain injury and leading to more or less severe problems in speaking, understanding, reading and/or writing. Papathanasiou and Coppens (2013) emphasize the fact that this impairment has an enormous impact on social functioning and quality of life, not only for the person with aphasia, but also for those of his/her surroundings. It is therefore not really surprising that the suddenly occurring and serious consequences of aphasia are the subject of a lot of books, films and theater performances.

(Auto)biographies and non-fiction

As far as **(auto)biographies** are concerned, it may seem strange that individuals who struggle with oral and written language, feel the need to write down the story of their illness. However several patient stories have been published, written by the person with aphasia him or herself, sometimes with some assistance of a relative or therapist. Some of these memoirs can be especially helpful for fellow-sufferers on their road to recovery from aphasia, but also for family or caregivers. Personal stories can help make this condition human and to create understanding, more than any textbook on aphasia can. We describe some examples.

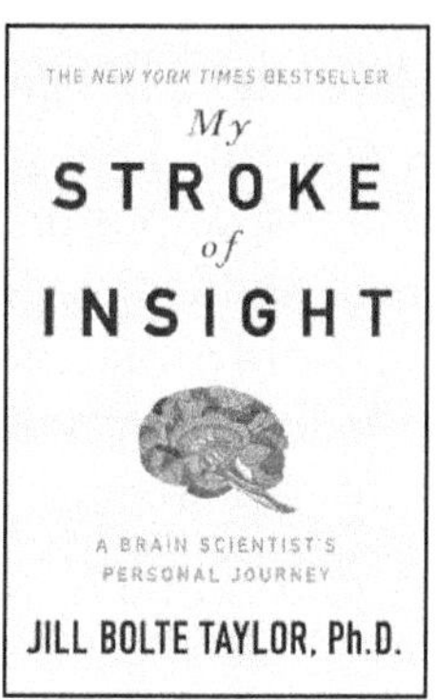

'*My stroke of insight*' was written by Jill Bolte Taylor (2008). Being a well-known brain scientist herself, she was only 37 years old when one of her brain arteries collapsed. Amazed she saw how her brain failed her, how she could no longer talk, walk, read or write and how she lost the memories of her former life.

In her autobiography she describes how she largely recovered from her stroke. The book also provides some guidelines for people who have had similar experiences and offers some insight into how the human brain works.

Lauren Marks was only 27 years old, when an aneurysm ruptured in her brain. She woke up in a hospital with serious deficiencies to her reading, speaking, and writing abilities, and a diagnosis unfamiliar to her: aphasia. Soon after, she began writing a journal, to chronicle her year following the rupture. The book *'A Stitch of Time'* was the result. She describes how she had to relearn and re-experience many of the things we take for granted—reading a book, understanding idioms,... This story has been reviewed as deeply personal and powerful, an unforgettable journey of self-discovery, resilience, and hope.

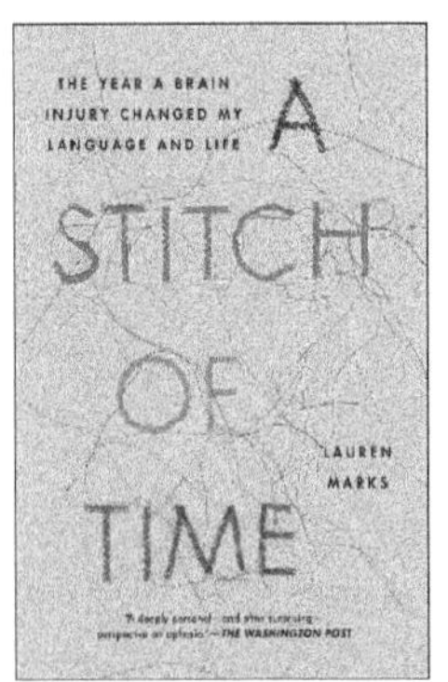

'A mind of my own. Memoir of recovery from Aphasia', written by Harrianne Mills (2004), describes the true story of the recovery from a traumatic brain injury following a motorcycle accident in Greece. With much more than fractures and physical complaints, this professor in classical history also loses what is most important for her, namely her speech and language skills. When she wakes up from coma, she even doesn't recognize her relatives. Follows a description of her recovery trajectory, using diary excerpts, medical reports and letters, thus shedding light on the problems she encounters in

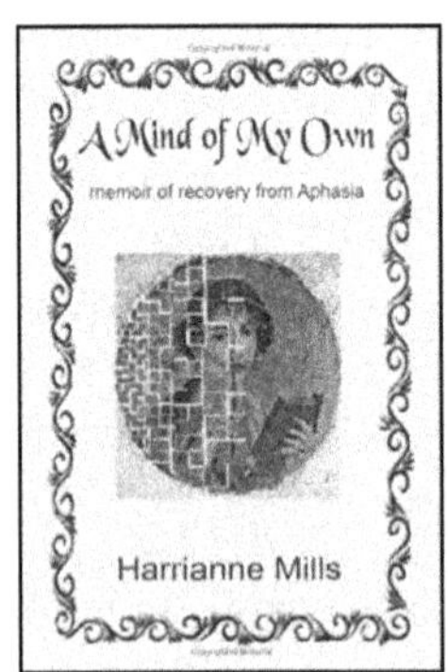

becoming a fully-fledged person again from different perspectives.

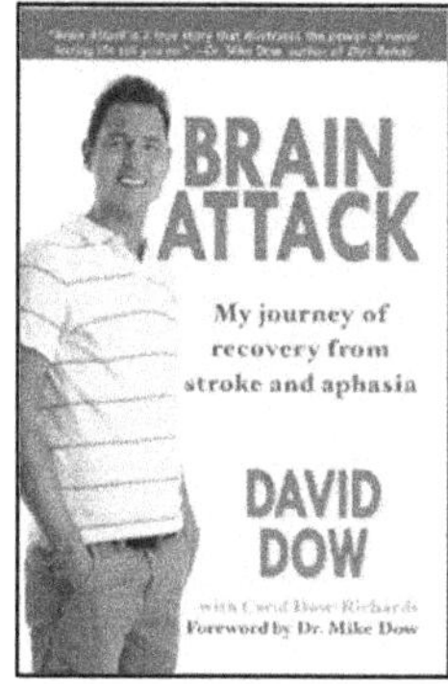

David Dow was only ten years old when his life suddenly changed drastically due to a stroke. He had a paralysis on his right side and was unable to speak, write and read due to aphasia. In his book *'Brain Attack: my journey of recovery from stroke and aphasia'* (2013), he describes his own story plainly. Later Dow became an advocate for people suffering from stroke and aphasia. He also co-authored *'ARC's Guide to Living with Aphasia: Practical Advice for People with Aphasia & Their Loved Ones'* (Dow-Richards, Anderson, Dow & Eaton, 2020),

In December, 2001, the HIV virus caused a serious brain infection in the Dutch art collector and writer Han Nefkens (°1954). He is in a coma for weeks and when he wakes up it turns out that he has aphasia: he cannot speak or read and no longer understands language. But he can no longer perform daily activities such as eating or walking alone either. Pieces from his past are inaccessible.
Nefkens describes in the book *'De gevlogen vogel'* (The Flown Bird) his slow recovery during the following five years, how he had to learn inch by inch what had been so natural before: eating, walking, speaking, reading and writing. Initially he sees and understands only small pieces, no wholes, no connections, no feelings of others. Without his memories, his life is a chaos of loose grains of sand. He feels like a different person. Only the moment is real, every moment again. It is a recovery with many obstacles and problems, for himself and especially for his partner. He describes his regained life with a lot of humor, in short pieces of one or a few pages. We quote a short excerpt from this book:

"Eating a cheese sandwich was an impossible task: not only did I lack the strength to cut the bread and bring the fork to my mouth, I also didn't know how to do it. But all of that was nothing compared to the impotence I felt because the words were hiding in my head. I knew they were somewhere, but I couldn't reach them - the harder I searched, the more I got lost. The words that did emerge were not attached to an image, they were words without meaning, as if they came from a language I did not speak. "Wednesday" meant the same as "buttermilk", "pillowcase" was "strawberry jam". My mind was empty. Every now and then I heard an echo, but I did not know what it was an echo of. (pp. 15-16).

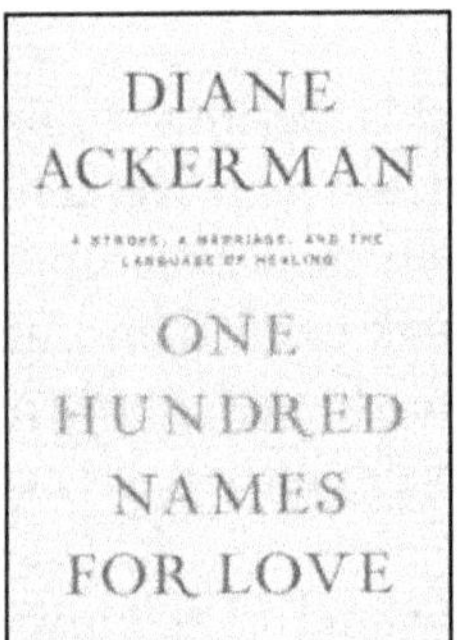

Some revealing biographies on aphasia, written by relatives, are '*One hundred names for love*' by Diane Ackerman(2011) and '*The man who lost his language. A case of aphasia*' by Sheila Hale.

In the book '*One hundred names for love*', the American Diane Ackerman describes the medical history of her husband Paul West, an exceptionally talented word artist and intellectual, who suffered a serious stroke. When he regained consciousness he was found to have aphasia and could only utter one syllable, "mem". Standard therapies proved unsuccessful, but Diane Ackerman found that by combining their mutual familiarity with each other and her own knowledge of language and of the brain, she could trace her husband back to the world of words.

'The Man who Lost His Language' is a unique exploration of what aphasia is and at the same time a testimony to the resilience of love. In 1992 Sir John Hale, a British historian and translator, who was famous for his Renaissance studies, suffers a severe stroke that affects his ability to walk, speak, and write. His wife Sheila, herself a distinguished travel writer and journalist, seeks out all available medical information about his condition and how it could be improved. The latest, revised version of this book contains an additional chapter describing the most recent scientific and medical developments. This personal account of a couple's experiences is of interest to anyone wishing to learn more about aphasia and related conditions. In reviews this book has been described as a unique exploration of aphasia from the personal perspective of a couple coming to terms with its challenges and adapting to life after a debilitating stroke. John Hale died in 1999.

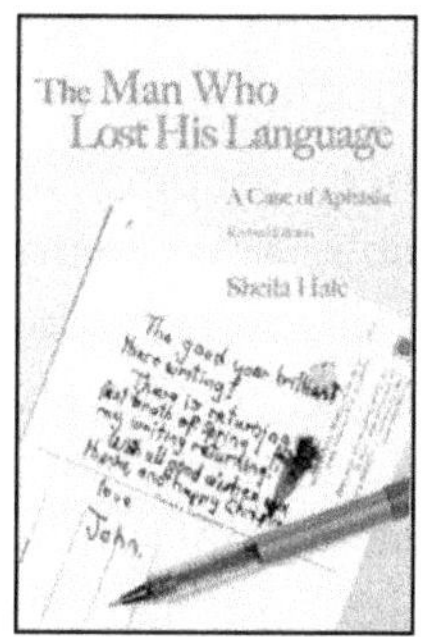

Fictional literature

In **classic** French **literature** we find some descriptions of people suffering from aphasia in the novels *'Thérèse Raquin'* (1867) and *'La Terre'* (1887) by Emile Zola. In the first book Thérèse's aunt suffers from a stroke, leading to a complete loss of her language facilities. In his monograph *'De l'aphasie et de ses diverses formes'* (Aphasia and its various forms, 1889), the author Désiré Bernard indicates that Zola was about the only writer in that time who described aphasia with a certain degree of clinical accuracy.

We quote a short excerpt:

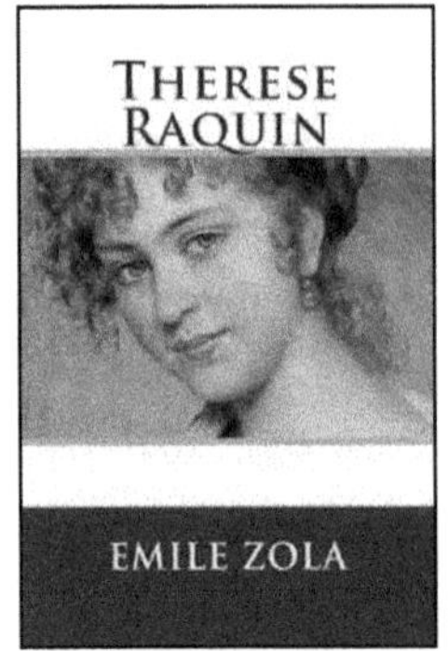

"One night, while she was talking quietly with Thérèse and Laurent, she paused in the middle of a sentence, gasping for breath, feeling like she was being strangled. She tried to call for help, but could only make a few hoarse noises. Her tongue had turned to stone. Her hands and feet stiffened. She was dumbfounded and motionless. Thérèse and Laurent stood up, startled as if by a bolt of thunder, which hit this woman in less than five seconds. When she froze and looked at them with a pleading look, they bombarded her with questions to find out the cause of her suffering. She couldn't answer and kept looking at them with a look of deep fear. Then they realized that there was nothing left for them but a body, a body that was half alive and could see and hear them but could not speak" (p. 315-316)

When Mrs. Raquin later witnesses a quarrel between Thérèse and Laurent, in which they accuse each other of being responsible for the murder of her son, she tries to communicate this crime to two visitors. With superhuman effort, she manages to take a pen, with the intention of writing "Thérèse et Laurent ont tué Camille" (Thérèse and Laurent have murdered Camille), but her strength gives way and she gets stuck with "Thérèse et Laurent ont t...". The visitors become frustrated and interpret her message as "Thérèse et Laurent ont été très bien pour moi" (Thérèse and Laurent have been good to me). As a result, her chance to expose their crime has been lost.

The novella *'La Terre'*, which Zola himself considered his masterpiece, also mentions a number of cases of apoplexy or bruising in the brain, two of which result in a (temporary) loss of language ability (Eagle, 2014) . Thus is described the case of one Mouche, who is found affected by "une attaque d'apoplexie" (brain apoplexy). When he is brought home and his daughter Lise sees the face of her father, one half of which is completely deformed, she says, “Father, say something, please. What the hell is going on? It's in your head, isn't it, and that's why you can't say anything ”. This last question clearly indicates that Zola was well aware that language faculty was localized in the brain and not in the organs of speech, and thus may have been aware of the findings and publications of Paul Broca, the father of modern aphasiology, who showed in 1861 that language capacity was located in the frontal lobe of the language-dominant hemisphere (in right handed persons usually the left).

Marcel Proust (1871-1922), widely known for his novel cycle *‘A la recherche du temps perdu’* (In search of time lost), should not be reminded of the fragility of language and the devastating effects of a brain hemorrhage. After all, his father died in 1903 of a stroke. He was a physician who himself researched and published on neurological and, more specifically, aphasic disorders. Two years later, Proust’s mother became paralyzed and she developed sudden aphasia as a complication of renal failure (Eagle, 2014). She passed away two days later. It is well known that Proust based the description of Marcel's grandmother's illness and death in the "Recherche-cycle" on the condition of his own mother during the last days of her life. He writes that, as a result of kidney failure, first the grandmother's vision begins to deteriorate, then her hearing, her mobility and finally her speech:

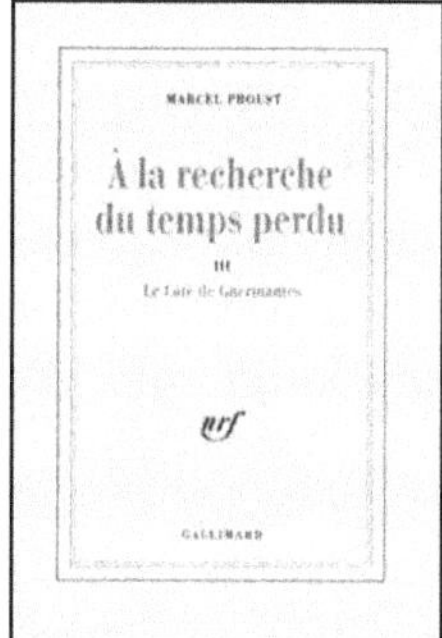

> “Her pain decreased, but her speech impediment increased. We were forced to ask her to repeat almost everything she said. And when she realized that we could no longer understand her, she gave up her attempts to speak and lay there in complete silence ”.

From the day his mother died, Proust had a pathological fear of losing his ability to speak as well. This "aphasia phobia" was exacerbated when in 1917 the writer began to show symptoms of amnesia, facial paralysis and speech disorders. His speaking became dragging, probably due to the abuse of barbiturates. He noticed more and more slips of the tongue and found that it was difficult or impossible to pronounce certain words. His own experiences found their way into the description of some characters from the 'Recherche'- cycle. The writings about aphasia by his father, Adrien Proust (including '*De l'aphasie*' (Aphasia, 1872), may have been an important source of inspiration for son Marcel. He thus accurately describes the disease of a certain Baron de Charlus. This baron ends up in a kind of linguistic waterfall and turns from the "greatest chatterer in the world" into a frail aphasic, who can only "pronounce a few words with difficulty and incorrectly" (Eagle, 2014).

In English classic literature we also find some references to persons suffering from aphasia (Sainsbury, Wyles & Tillard, 2012). An example can be found in Charles Dickens' book '*Bleak house*', in which Sir Leicester Dedlock suffers from a stroke and can't express himself no longer using spoken language. We cite:

> "He fell down, this morning, a handsome stately gentleman, somewhat infirm, but of a fine presence, and with a well-filled face. Now he lies upon his bed, an aged man with sunken cheeks, the decrepit shadow of himself. His voice was rich and mellow and he had so long been thoroughly persuaded of the weight and import to mankind of any word he said that his words really had come to sound as if there were something in them. But now he can only whisper, and what he whispers sounds like what it is—mere jumble and jargon.

After vainly trying to make himself understood in speech, he makes signs for a pencil. So inexpressively that they cannot at first understand him; it is his old housekeeper who makes out what he wants and brings in a slate ... . After pausing for some time, he slowly scrawls upon it in a hand that is not his, 'Chesney Wold[1]?' (BH,691)

George Eliot, pseudonym for Mary Anne Evans, describes in 'The mill on the Floss' how a certain Mr Tulliver gets in financial troubles and has a stroke while returning home. Also a citation:

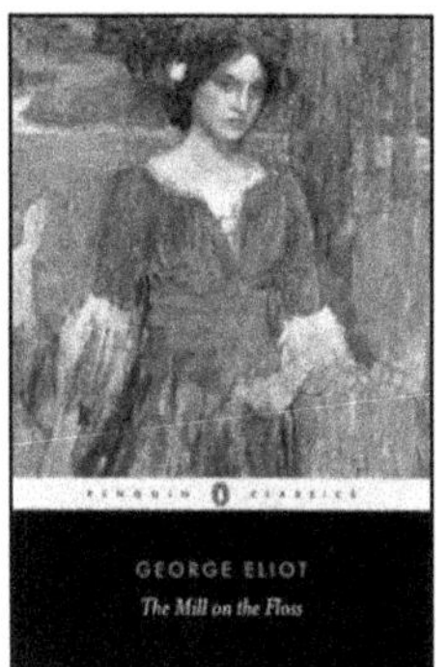

"Mr Tulliver's own wagoner found him lying by the roadside, with an open letter near him ... he had become conscious, and after vague, vacant looks around him, had muttered something about 'a letter'. His only words were 'a letter' and 'the little wench' (referring to his favourite Maggie). He repeated the words from time to time, appearing entirely unconscious of everything except this one importunate want, and giving no sign of knowing his wife or anyone else".

In his novel '*War and Peace*' (1869), the well-known Russian author Leo Tolstoy draws a picture of Prince Bolkonsky. The information provided allows us to identify the terminal illness of the prince as a brain stem haemorrhage. His left side is paralysed and his speech is limited to inarticulate mumbling (Albin, 1990). For more details we refer to Sainsbury, Wyles and Tillard (2012).

In more recent literature we find a person showing aphasia in the 2019 French novel '*Les Gratitudes*' by Delphine de Vigan (2019). She describes an elderly woman who loses her language

---

[1] Chesney Wold is the name of the estate where Sir Dedlock lives

progressively. This book has very recently been translated into English as *'Gratitude'* (2021).

Another French book about the effects of stroke has been written by Georges Simenon, world famous for his 'Inspector Maigret'-series. In *'The Bells of Bicêtre'* the author analyses the effect of a stroke on a man in the prime of his life. René Maugras has risen from obscurity to being a publisher of a highly influential Paris newspaper. Then suddenly he finds himself in a Paris hospital, speechless and paralyzed, yet surprisingly clear of mind. In the book we follow his slow recovery, surrounded by his physician friend Besson, his nurses, and various visitors at the Hospital of Bicêtre in the southern suburbs of Paris. Maugras passively undergoes treatment day after day, recalling his youth, his friends, his work, his first wife and his second wife in a whirlpool of emotions. This brilliant book was also published with the title *'The patient'*.

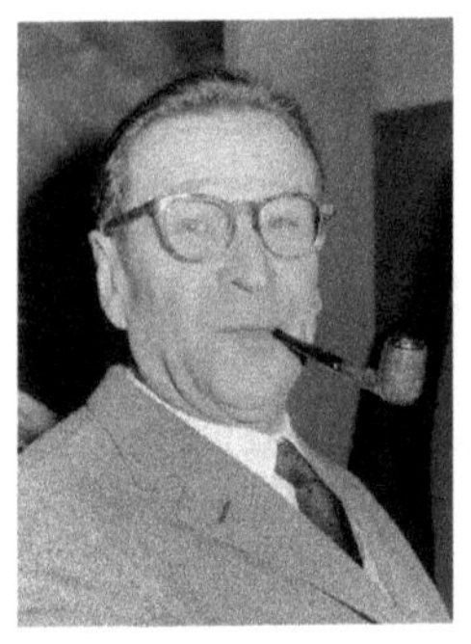

'*Speechless*', a novel written by Kim Fielding (2012) also features a person with aphasia. In this book, the protagonist Travis Miller has a dull job, a cat named Elwood, and a rather pathetic love life. The only ray of hope in his life is the handsome guitarist, whom he sometimes passes by on the way home from work. But when he finally finds the courage to address the man, he finds out that this former writer is suffering from aphasia: the man called Drew can understand everything Travis is telling him, but cannot speak or write. The two men befriend, which ends in a romance. But the communication problem is just one of the challenges they have to face.

'*Sprakeloos*', by the Belgian author Tom Lanoye and in English also translated as '*Speechless*' is a touching memoir about the final years of the writer's mother.

After a stroke, she, who is a butcher's wife and an obsessive amateur actress, becomes aphasic. Slowly but inevitably she loses her ability to speak and she is more and more unable to communicate with her loved ones. In the book, Lanoye draws up a multiple balance: of his colourful youth in a working-class neighbourhood, of his struggle with love, of his role as a writer, of his conflicts with the little mother diva, of the courageous struggle that his mother wages and in which it goes down irretrievably, unreasonably and speechless, and from the lasting anger and pain that this produces. Speechless is a poignant ode to his mother. As the writer describes it: 'She lost first her speech, then her dignity, then her heartbeat' (p. 7.).

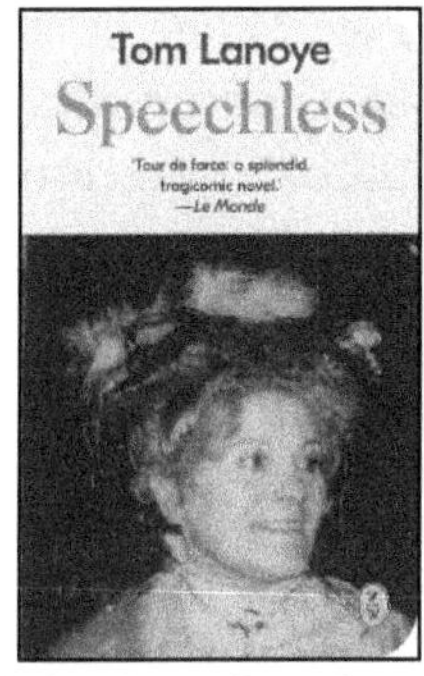

In the second part, *'The Wat*er *Rituals*', of the thrilling detective trilogy *'The White City*' by the Spanish Eva García Sáenz de Urturi, the main character, Inspector Unai López de Ayala, recovers from a gunshot wound that has left him with aphasia. His inability to speak frustrates him and makes it very difficult for him to do his job as he was used to. In the first instance, this forces him to communicate with word processing using a tablet for the time being.

Film and theater

Let's turn to the **theater** first. In July 1988, just over a year before his death, Samuel Beckett, the famous playwright and 1969 Nobel Prize winner, fell down in his kitchen and was found unconscious. Medical examinations were inconclusive. He was thought to have either had a stroke or suffered from Parkinson's disease, although he did not exhibit the typical hand tremor. The exact cause of his neurological disorder may be uncertain, but its consequence was clear: Beckett experienced a temporary but severely limiting aphasia (Salisbury, 2008).

As his speaking and writing skills slowly returned, he began to work at the Hôpital Pasteur in Paris on a poem entitled *'Comment Dire'*, later translated into English as '*What is the word*'. Packed with repetitions, abrupt omissions, compulsive reiterations, which seem to emerge from a kind of mysterious no man's land between the voluntary and the involuntary, this poem can be seen as a reflection of Beckett's aphasia and as a compulsive word search, in a sort of telegraphic style.

We cite a small fragment:

> *folly -*
> *folly for to -*
> *for to -*
> *what is the word -*
> *folly from this -*
> *all this -*
> *folly from all this -*
> *given - ...*

Theater critic Ruby Cohn read the poem in several different versions and noticed a connection with the hesitant nature, which is typical of aphasic speech. She immediately thought of the actor and theater-maker Joe Chaikin, who had been performing Beckett's work since the 1960s, but who suffered from aphasia since 1984 after a stroke complicating his third open-heart surgery. Since Chaikin did not know French, Cohn asked Beckett to translate the poem, but he couldn't even remember writing it. After she sent him a copy, he made a translation, which he dedicated to Joe Chaikin. Moreover, it was also the last work that Beckett wrote.

Despite his aphasia, Chaikin continued to act, albeit with adapted lyrics. In 1995 he retired from acting with some of Beckett's latest lyrics: 'Texts for nothing', 'Hey Joe' and the aforementioned 'What is the word'. The farewell tour also took him to Belgium and in a newspaper, dating from February, 1995, the journalist Geert Sels describes his meeting with Joe Chaikin, clearly showing the uncomfortable attitude a layman has towards a person with aphasia.

We quote an excerpt from the newspaper article:

> "We face each other and exchange a long glance. No words, they don't come that quickly. Thoughts all the more. So this is Joe Chaikin. Can I start a conversation with him right away, or would he not understand me? Should I speak loudly, use simple words, or articulate clearly so that he can read my lips? I hope to read the correct answer from his face. Inquisitive, he tilts his head a little, his eyes a question. I can't help but think of the puppy we once had at home. He may be wary. Anxious at having to start a language battle in a moment. Fortunately, there are ways discomfort can be covered up. So we shake hands and exchange a few words of greeting. He mumbles, so do I.
> Still not all consonants come out smoothly and the syntax of his sentences has been reduced to the bare necessities. But at least he speaks. "Brains is bad. Mess up words", he says".

We quote another excerpt from one of Beckett's texts, which Chaikin brought to the stage, and which aptly describes the loss of language, being the actor's working tool:

> *Powerful grasp of language you had...*
> *Flint glass...*
> *You could have listened to it for ever*
> *And now this...*
> *Squeezed down to this*
> *How much longer would you say?*
> *Till the whisper?*
> *You know, when you can't hear the words*
> *Just the odd one here and there*

That is the worst, isn't it Joe

(from Hey Joe, Samuel Becket)

Chaikin died in 2003 at the age of 67.

We found a number of English language films, often **documentaries**, devoted to the problem of aphasia. In many cases it concerns testimonials from people who have been affected by the condition and who tell their own story, alone or with the help of loved ones and/or therapists.

'*The Possibilities Are Endless*' (2014) is a BBC music documentary and the third film by Edward Lovelace and James Hall about Scottish singer-songwriter Edwyn Collins. He made a name for himself with the post-punk band 'Orange Juice' and also as a songwriter with hits such as 'Rip it up' and 'A girl like you'. But in February 2005, Collins suffered a brain hemorrhage that was so severe that the doctors initially feared he would not survive. He eventually made it, but he had suffered serious brain damage. He had lost his ability to speak and the only two things he could say were "Grace Maxwell," his wife's name, and "the possibilities are endless".

The film starts with a short clip of a talk show performance at the moment Edwyn was still healthy. Then fragments of his memories follow in an attempt to recall his life, as it was before that near-fatal brain hemorrhage. Together with his wife and manager Grace, Collins tells in a voice-over about the long road to recovery. This story is beautifully colored with fragments of old, but also of recent performances and the preparations for them, and with breathtaking images of the Scottish landscape. Furthermore, the film contains a mix of realistic images and scenes in which his son Will reenacts how his father met his mother in his early years - a story that beautifully sketches the intimate and strong bond between these two persons[2].

'After Words' is a documentary, directed by Jerome Kaplan and Vincent Straggas in 2003. The aim of the film was to shed light on the disorder 'aphasia' through the stories of members of the Aphasia Community Group of Boston (ACG) , a self-help group for people affected by the condition. These individuals are filmed in their home environment, as well as in their community, at work or during group meetings. A number of famous persons who have suffered stroke and aphasia are also brought up, such as the above mentioned actor Joseph Chaikin, Julie Harris and Patricia Neal, actress and for some time the wife of writer Roald Dahl.

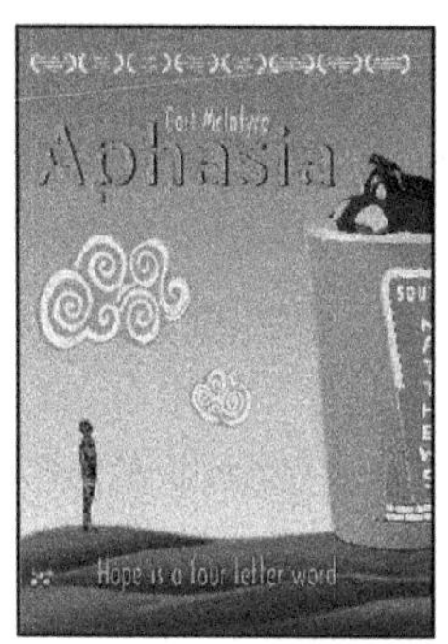

Directed by Jim Gloster, the film *'Aphasia'* (2010) tells the story of actor Carl McIntyre, who survived a severe brain hemorrhage in 2005 and, as a consequence, was unable to speak, read and write. Prior to the stroke, Carl was a successful film, television and theater actor. The language difficulties he exhibits as a person with aphasia are of course a serious obstacle in the pursuit of his career, but they do not interfere with his ability to portray human emotions and interactions. In the film *'Aphasia'*, Carl plays himself and conveys his life story with incredible nuance. A story with both humor and perseverance. More information on this film and fragments of interviews with the actor can be found on the internet[3].

'Picturing Aphasia' is a short documentary film directed by Mores McWreath and released in 2006. Its purpose is to help people recently affected by aphasia understand that

---

[2] For a trailer, see: https://www.youtube.com/watch?v=9wbknwieX0Q

[3] See: https://www.aphasiathemovie.com/Aphasia_Project/About_Carl.html

rehabilitation is not only possible but also desirable. The film explores the boundaries between visual and non-visual language. Four people talk about their lives with aphasia. Their stories are supported and illustrated by means of drawings, which leads to a very nice result. A trailer can be also be found on YouTube[4].

When Sophie Salveson was 19 years old, she had a life filled with friends, family, musical theater and travel. Now, at the age of 24, her life still revolves around her loved ones and the stage, but there is an important difference, which is aphasia. A stroke at the age of 19 suddenly changed her life path. The short film *'Still Sophie'* (2016, directed by Caroline Knight) shows how her communication disorders affect her daily life. The "National Aphasia Association" has sponsored this film, which has already won a number of awards. Sophie is portrayed as an honest, cheerful young woman with a beautiful singing voice. The film proves that despite the struggle to find words, Sophie is still the same person with the same desire for love.

The excellent documentary *'My Beautiful Broken Brain'* dates from 2014. This film traces the emotional journey of Londoner Lotje Sodderland, who suffered a brain hemorrhage in 2011 when she was only 34 years old. She could no longer read, write and talk coherently. It focuses on the day-to-day challenges her aphasia and apraxia bring along, as well as on a number of other issues she experiences, such as memory disorders, sensory changes, fatigue and frustration. Her rehabilitation process includes physiotherapy, occupational therapy, speech therapy and psychiatric support. From the beginning of her condition, even when she was still

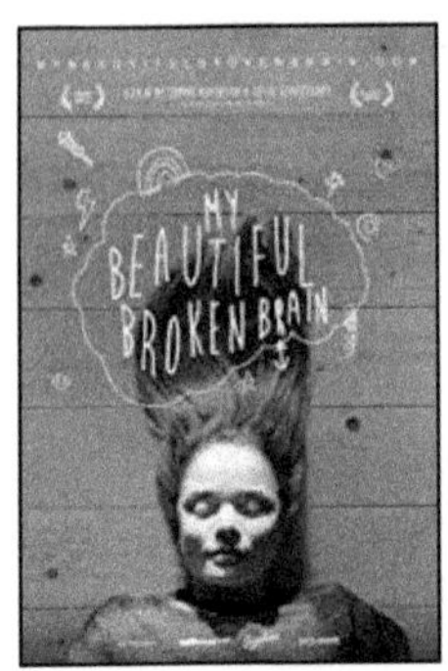

[4] Trailer of Picturing Aphasia: https://www.youtube.com/watch?v=vyx4HVLgo7o

in hospital, she started filming herself with her smartphone. This self-made footage has been used extensively for the film.

In the 1991 **fiction film** *'Regarding Henry'* directed by Mike Nichols, Harrison Ford plays the role of Henry Turner. This is a ruthless lawyer, whose life is completely turned upside down when he is shot in the head during a robbery. Thanks to extensive brain surgery, he survives this incident, but he is left with very serious brain damage and has to learn everything again: to walk, to talk and to function normally. He also has memory disorders and has to learn to adapt to his personal and family life. The film was shot at Burke Rehabilitation Hospital in White Plains near New York. It provides an interesting picture and insight into how speech therapists work with adult patients, who have suffered serious brain damage.

References chapter 1

Ackerman, D. (2011). *One hundred names for love*. Ww Norton & Co, New York.

Albin, R.L. (1990) The death of Nicholas Bolkonski. Neurology in Tolstoy's War and Peace. *Arch Neurology*, 47(2):225-6.

De Vigan, D. (2019). *Les Gratitudes*. Editions J.C. Lattès, Paris.

De Vigan, D. (2021). *Gratitude*. Bloomsbury publishing, London.

Dickens, C. (2011). *Bleak House*. Penguin books Ltd., London

Dow, D. (2013) *Brain Attack: My Journey of Recovery From Stroke and Aphasia*. Speechless Publishing Group, s.l.

Dow-Richards, C. Anderson, A., Dow, D. & Eaton, T. (2020). *ARC's Guide to Living with Aphasia: Practical Advice for People with Aphasia & Their Loved Ones*. Aphasia Recovery Connection, Henderson, Nevada.

Eagle, C. (2014). *Dysfluencies. On Speech Disorders in Modern Literature*. Bloomsbury, New York/London.

Eliot, G. (2005). *The Mill on the Floss*. Penguin books, London.
Fielding, K. (2012) *Speechless*. Dreamspinner Press, Tallahassee, Florida.
Hale, S. (2007). *The Man Who Lost his Language: A Case of Aphasia*. Jessica Kingsley Publishers, London.
Lanoye, T. (2016). *Speechless*. World editions, New York/London.
Marks, L. (2017). *A Stitch of Time*. Simon & Schuster, New-York.
Mills, H. (2004). *A mind of my own. Memoir of recovery from aphasia*. Uitgeverij Authorhouse, Bloomington.
Nefkens, H. (2008). *De gevlogen vogel. Notities over een herwonnen leven*. Atlas, Amsterdam/Antwerpen.
Papathanasiou, I., Coppens, P. (2013). Aphasia and related communications disorders: basic concepts and operational definitions. In Papathanasiou, I., Coppens, P., Potagas, C. (Ed.). *Aphasia and related communications disorders*, Jones & Bartlett, Burlington.
Proust, M. (1907-1922). *A la recherche du temps perdu*. Gallimard, Paris.
Sainsbury, R., Wyles, C., Tillard, G. (2012). Neurological speech deficits as plot devices in novels. *Journal of the Royal Society of Medicine*, 105: 530–534. DOI 10.1258/jrsm.2012.120040
Salisbury, L. (2008). 'What Is the Word': Beckett's Aphasic Modernism. *Journal of Beckett Studies*, 17 (1-2); 78-126.
Simenon, G. (1965). *The Bells of Bicêtre*. Signet, New York.
Taylor, J.B. (2009). *My stroke of insight. A brain scientist's personal journey*. Hodder & Stoughton, London.
Tolstoj, L. (1869). *War and Peace*. The Russian Messenger, Moscow
Williams, A. N. (2003). Cerebrovascular disease in Dumas' The count of Monte Cristo. *Journal of the Royal Society of Medicine*; August 2003; 96, 8; 412-414.
Zola, E. (1873). *Thérèse Raquin*. Editions L'Artiste. Paris
Zola, E. (1887). *La Terre*. Editions Charpentier, Paris.

Chapter 2: Locked-in syndrome

Locked-in syndrome (LIS) is a rare neurological condition caused by brain stem injury. A blood clot gets stuck in the brain stem in such a way that stimuli are no longer transferred. As a result, all motor functions, including talking and swallowing, are blocked and the affected person becomes completely paralyzed. However, the intellectual and spiritual possibilities remain intact, so that thinking, fantasizing and dreaming remain possible. Literally locked-in means "locked up in your own body". In a 'classic' or complete locked-in condition only eye movements are preserved, so that the person concerned can only communicate by blinking the eyes (Snoeys, Van Hoof & Manders, 2013).

(Auto)biographies and non-fiction

We found some very inspiring **autobiographies** from persons with LIS. In the Dutch speaking regions Roland Boulengier, a former teacher of English, wrote four books about his condition and the way he experienced it: '*De eenzame stilte*' (The lonely silence, 2001), '*Dat andere leven*' (That other live, 2005), '*PAB-geassisteerd leven. De wereld van een locked-in*' (Assisted live, the world of locked-in, 2007) and '*Verlengingen*' (Extensions, 2009). In this last book the author describes how he was floating between life and death for several days due to aspiration pneumonia and how he struggled to recover.

In '*Het neusgatenperspectief*' (The nostril perspective, 1999), also written in Dutch, the former theater technician Paul Antipoff describes how he developed a locked-in condition when on vacation in Africa in August 1993. Antipoff suddenly got neck pain, nausea and fever. The next morning he could no longer stand on his feet and a day later he was completely paralyzed, probably from an infection with an as yet unknown virus. As a result of progressive paralysis, his breathing stopped and he went into a sub-comatose state. He was repatriated to Belgium in a very critical condition. Ten days later he awoke in a hospital in Brussels. He could no longer move, no longer speak, no longer breathe. A few years later he started writing down his emotions and experiences, at first just for himself. Then the idea grew to publish a book about that fight with oneself, the medical world and its environment. The question is how can you continue to live in such a strange situation? Penetrating and in sometimes almost poetic language, Antipoff talks in 'The nostril perspective' about the loss of self-esteem, the breakdown of his relationship and a new future he has to build. His criticism on the medical services is also often harsh. He wrote this interesting document letter by letter using a laser beam mounted on a spectacle frame from the wheelchair user's 'nostril perspective'.

Perhaps the best-known autobiographical book about LIS is written by the Frenchman Jean-Dominique Bauby, entitled *'le Scaphandre et le Papillon'* (1997), translated into English as *'The diving bell and the butterfly'*. The book was also made into a compelling and moving film in 2007, directed by Julian Schnabel (see below).

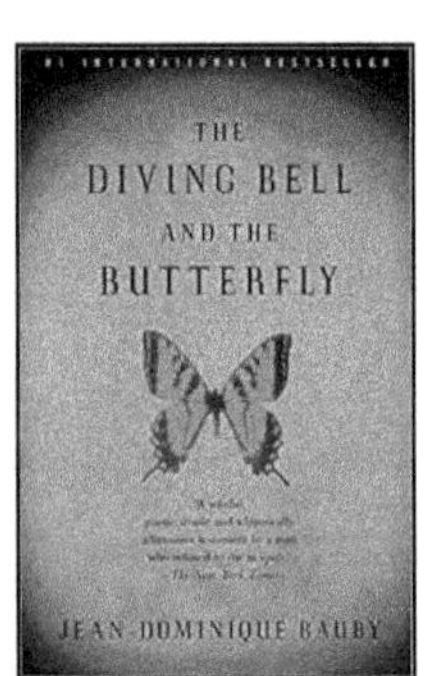

Bauby was editor-in-chief of the fashion magazine 'Elle' when, at the age of 43, he got struck by a brain stem haemorrhage and ended up in a locked-in condition. He wrote his autobiographical book by means of eye blinking and using a special alphabet system, developed by his speech therapist.
We cite a small fragment from the prologue:

> Through the frayed curtain at my window, a wan glow announces the break of day. My heels hurt, my head weighs a ton, and something like a giant invisible diving bell holds my whole body prisoner. My room emerges slowly from the gloom. (....)

> No need to wonder very long where I am, or to recall that the life I once knew was snuffed out Friday, the eighth of December, last year. Up until then, I had never even heard of the brain stem. I've since learned that it is an essential component of our internal computer, the inseparable link between the brain and the spinal cord. I was brutally introduced to this vital piece of anatomy when a cerebrovascular accident took my brainstem out of action. In the past, it was known as a "massive stroke," and you simply died. But improved resuscitation techniques have now prolonged and refined the agony. You survive, but you survive with what is so aptly known as "locked-in syndrome." Paralyzed from head to toe, the patient, his mind intact, is imprisoned inside his own body, unable to speak or move. In my case, blinking my left eyelid is my only means of communication. (p. 9)

Bauby died only a few days after his book was published.

'Look up for Yes' (1988) written by Julia Tavalaro (with the help of Richard Tayson) is the passionate and lucid story of a woman who woke up from a coma at the age of 32 after having experienced two strokes and couldn't speak no more. She also, like Bauby, became a prisoner in her own body from one moment to the next and she fell victim to what she considered to be the ignorant and cruel treatment of hospital staff, who did not pay attention to her and did not care that the 'plant' they refreshed and fed every day, was in reality a sensible and emotional woman. In this powerful document, Tavalaro describes the hell she endured as a defenseless patient and the liberating actions of two therapists, who took the time to realize that she was not ignorant, but brimming with intellect

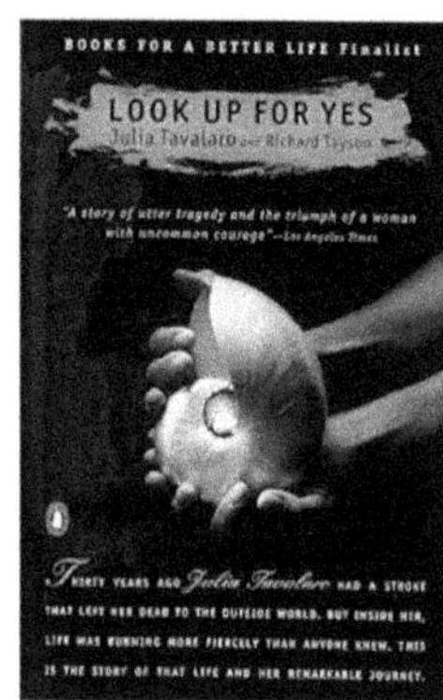

and life. She eventually managed to break through the isolation and very slowly regained her ability to communicate, using technological and therapeutic advancements, and even began to write poems and lyrics that harked back to her pre-stroke memories.

'*Putain de silence*', translated into English as '*Only the eyes say yes*' (2000), is the story of Philippe Vigand and his wife Stéphane. He was 32, she 28, they had two children and life went on. Then one of his blood vessels broke down and he woke up completely paralyzed after two months in a coma, making his medical history very similar to that of Bauby. His heart, lungs and brain were still working perfectly. A speech therapist was the first to realize that his brain was intact when he asked how much 2 x 2 was and Philippe blinked 4 times. It is their struggle against this ordeal, which Philippe and Stéphane each describe from their own point of view in this book through two complementary testimonies, what makes this an exceptional story. Stéphane is convinced that her husband has not become a 'plant' and is making every effort in the world to develop a communication method, first via a letter-pointing system, later with the help of a computer, after he regains control over the use of a finger.

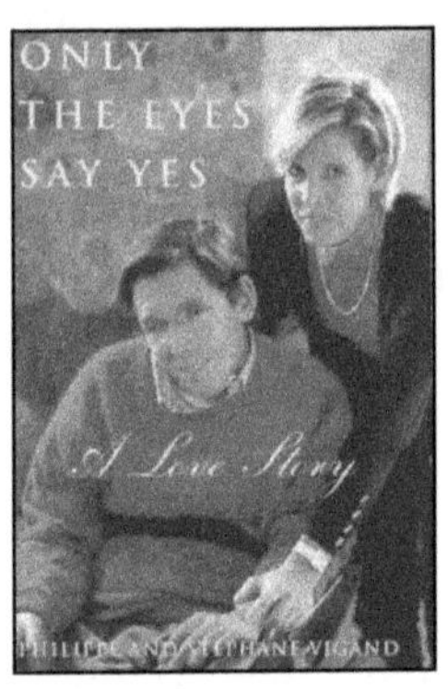

Another biography worth mentioning is '*Ghost boy*', written by the South African Martin Pistorius (° 1975). In this book he tells how he experienced the locked-in syndrome as a child. When he was twelve, everything started with a mysterious flu. Within a year and a half he was wheelchair bound and could no longer communicate.

Another biography worth mentioning is '*Ghost boy*', written by the South African Martin Pistorius (° 1975). In this book he tells how he experienced the locked-in syndrome as a child. When he was twelve, everything started with a mysterious flu. Within a year and a half he was wheelchair bound and could no longer communicate. He saw and heard everything, but no one noticed. The worst of his nightmares came true. Doctors thought of Martin to have the cognitive level of a newborn and he ended up in a care home for the disabled, where he became increasingly distant from the world. After eleven years, a therapist discovered that Martin did respond to stimuli. She paid attention to him, kept talking to him, and he began to communicate with his eyes. Thanks to her, he was able to free himself from his physical prison. 'Ghost Boy' is a moving book. As a reader you sympathize with Martin, with his inability to express himself. Martin Pistorius is currently able to communicate through a voice computer. He is married, lives in England and earns a living as an author and a web designer[5].

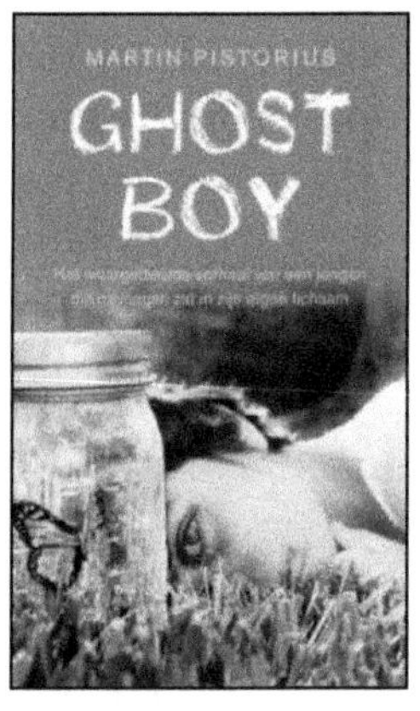

Fiction

In literary fiction we find some examples of characters suffering from locked-in syndrome. Alexandre Dumas gives an accurate description of the syndrome in his novel '*The count of Monte Cristo*' (Williams, 2003).
The condition of Monsieur Noirtier de Villefort is portrayed as if 'the soul is trapped in a body that no longer obeys its orders'.

[5] An inspiring Ted Talk by Martin Pistorius can be found on the internet: https://www.ted.com/talks/martin_pistorius_how_my_mind_came_back_to_life_and_no_one_knew

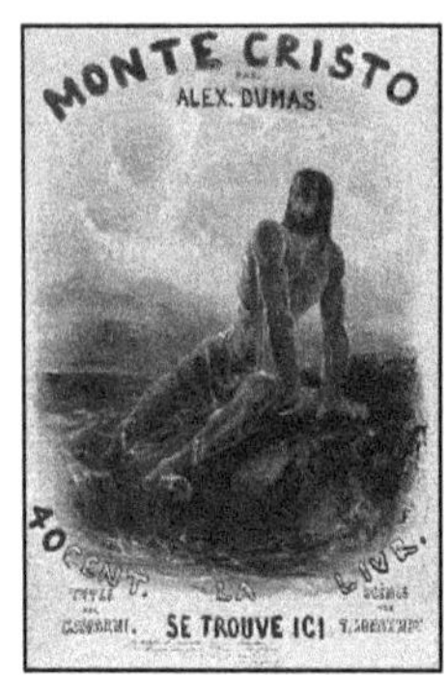

We cite a short fragment:

'Sight and hearing were the only two senses which, like two sparks, still lit up this human matter, already three quarters moulded for the tomb. Moreover only one of these two senses could reveal to the outside world the inner life, which animated this statue.... He was a corpse with living eyes, and at times, nothing could be more terrifying than this marble face out of which anger burned or joy shone.' (p. 564)

Although his intellectual capacities are intact, Noirtier de Villefort is unable to do anything physically. He is only able to communicate by blink of an eye, where one blink stands for "yes" and twice for "no". Dumas describes how his granddaughter Valentine teaches him how to use an alphabet card to spell words. This is about the same communication system that Jean-Dominique Bauby also used when writing his autobiography (see above).

The English author Charles Dickens mentions a case of LIS in his novel '*Little Dorrit*' (1857). He decribes how Mrs Clenman falls down and, from that moment on, is unable to move a finger and doesn't have the strength to utter one single word. Except from moving her eyes and shaking her head for yes and no, she lived on and died like a statue.

In more recent literature we find a description of a person with LIS in the book '*Agaat*' by the South African Marlene Van Niekerk. In this book, one of the characters, Milla Redelinghuys, can only speak with her eyes on her deathbed. Her black housekeeper Agaat, who takes care of her and on whom she depends, is the only one who understands her. While Milla ponders on her difficult life, Agaat reads Milla's diaries to her. In this way, a tragic past slowly comes to light, which simultaneously connects and dispels these two women.

In the original and exciting debut *'If I die before I wake'* (2018), Emily Koch portrays a narrator who fights against his own powerlessness and against time ticking away. Everyone is convinced that Alex is in a coma and will never wake up again. But in reality he hears everything being said around his hospital bed. He hears that his girlfriend is being talked about - she must forget about him and go on living. He overhears his family suggest that a mild death might be for the best. And then he learns that his accident may not have been an accident at all. Alex dives into his memories and torments his brain to discover who committed the assassination attempt. From the prison of his own body, he must find the answer before his treatment is stopped, and before anyone else gets killed, because Alex is not the only target .... The reader is drawn into a story full of subtlety, confusion, frustration and above all tension.

Film and music theater

Regarding films, we mentioned earlier that Jean-Dominique Bauby's autobiographical book and life story, *'The diving bell and the butterfly'*, was filmed in 2007 by director Julian Schnabel. Actor Matthieu Amalric empathizes with his role as a locked-in person incredibly well. The book is followed quite closely, with some very moving scenes. This film won awards at the Cannes Film Festival, the Golden Globes, the BAFTAs, and the César Awards, and received four Oscar nominations. Several critics later listed it as one of the best films of its decade.

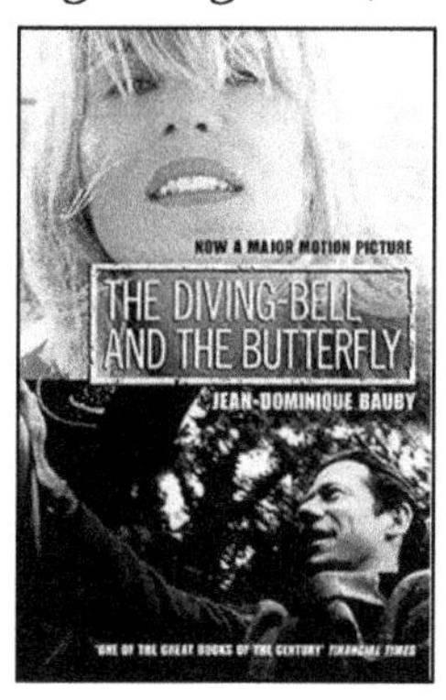

In the 2010 film *'Locked-in'* by director Suri Krishnamma, the protagonist's daughter becomes locked-in after a traffic accident. When everyone has already given up hope, she starts communicating with her father anyway. But something seems strange. Is she really communicating or is he going crazy?

On YouTube several videos about people in a locked-in condition can be found. There is the story of Nick Chisholm who suffered a stroke in 2000 after a rugby match, which caused LIS. The film shows his life at home, how his wife deals with his problems and also focusses on their social life, which of course has changed significantly. It's a brave portrait. The story of '*Mike and Tanya*' is also particularly poignant, as is the courageous "TED-X –talk" by the young the Finnish woman Kati Lepistö[6].

We didn't find theatrical performances in which people with LIS appear, but we did discover a 2014 opera production by Romeo Castellucci, based on Berlioz's French version of the opera '*Orpheus and Eurydice*", originally composed by Christoph Willibald Gluck. In this modern adaptation, the parallel is drawn between Eurydice, who is in the underworld and who Orfeo tries to bring back to the living, and the locked-in state in which Els, a young, 28 year old woman, ended up after a thrombosis. During the performance, video images of the young woman are continuously shown in the background, including some in which she is listening to the music with headphones and her reactions can be read based on the blinking of her eyes. Certain critics had mixed feelings about this: a clever find or a certain degree of voyeurism?

References chapter 2

Antipoff, P. (1999). *Het neusgatenperspectief.* Uitgeverij Epo, Berchem.

---

[6] https://www.youtube.com/watch?v=eB1rgvwQ_T8

Bauby, J-D (1997). *Le scaphandre et le Papillon*. Editions Robert Laffont, Paris.

Bauby, J-D (1998). *The Diving Bell and the Butterfly*. Vintage, New York.

Boulengier, R. (2001). *De eenzame stilte.* Drukkerij-Uitgeverij Demol.

Boulengier, R. (2005). *Dat andere leven. Thuis met locked-in.* SIG, Gijzegem.

Boulengier, R. (2007). *PAB-geassisteerd leren leven. De wereld van een locked-in*. SIG, Gijzegem.

Boulengier, R. (2009). *Verlengingen. Overleven als locked-in.* SIG, Gijzegem.

Dickens, C. (1857). *Little Doritt*. Bradbury and Evans, London.

Dumas, A. (2003). *The count of Monte Cristo. Penguin Classics,* London.

Koch, E. (2018). *If I die before I wake.* Harvill Secker, London.

Pistorius, M. (2016). *Ghost boy*. Simon & Schuster, New York.

Sainsbury, R., Wyles, C., Tillard, G. (2012). *Neurological speech deficits as plot devices in novels*. J R Soc Med , 105: 530–534. DOI 10.1258/jrsm.2012.120040

Snoeys, L., Vanhoof, G., Manders, E. (2013). Living with locked-in syndrome: an explorative study on health care situation, communication and quality of life. *Disability and Rehabilitation*, 35 (9), 713-718.

Tavalaro, J.(1988). *Look up for yes*. Penguin books, London.

Van Niekerk, Marlene (2006). *Agaat*, Tin House Books, Portland .

Vigand, Ph. & S. (2000). *Only the eyes say yes*. Arcade Publishing, New York (English language edition).

Williams, A. N. (2003). Cerebrovascular disease in Dumas' The count of Monte Cristo. Journal of the Royal Society of Medicine; August 2003; 96, 8; 412-414.

Chapter 3: Dysarthria

Dysarthria can be defined as a group of speech disorders that result from problems with muscle control (slackening, slowing down or reduced coordination) and is caused by an injury to the central or peripheral nervous system. Disturbances can occur in one or more basic processes of speech: breathing, use of voice, resonance, articulation and/or prosody (Darley, Aronson & Brown, 1975). Dysarthria can occur in very different forms and degrees, ranging from a mildly lingering speech to complete unintelligibility and even total inability to speak. In the latter case, one usually speaks of anarthria. It could be argued that the locked-in syndrome (see chapter 2) usually also gives rise to anarthria.

We noticed that most of the stories and films, as well as children's and youth books, featuring persons with dysarthria, are related to cases of Cerebral Palsy (CP) and, in adults and to a lesser extent, to Amyotrophic Lateral Sclerosis (ALS), also often called Lou Gehrig's disease, after the famous baseball player who was diagnosed with it.

In the examples that we will discuss, there are many people who are forced to make do with certain forms of alternative and/or augmentative communication (AAC).

(Auto)biographies and non-fiction

One of the best-known persons, who first showed dysarthria and later evolved into anarthria, is the late genius scientist Stephen Hawking. In 1962, at the age of 20, during the last months he spent at Oxford University, Hawking found himself becoming increasingly clumsy, slurred in his speech, falling over and bumping into things. Amyotrophic lateral sclerosis (ALS) was diagnosed. Despite his illness, he obtained his doctoral degree, but he soon ended up in a wheelchair. In the summer of 1985, Hawking contracted life-threatening pneumonia. He was admitted to intensive care and had to be kept alive with machines. Ultimately, a tracheotomy had to be performed, as a result of which his voice, already severely weakened by dysarthria, was now permanently lost. From now on, Hawking could only communicate through his wife, who pointed out the letters, while Hawking moved his eyebrows

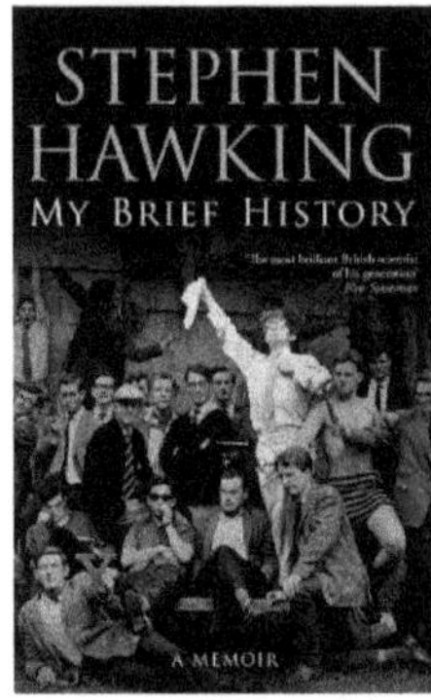

when she was on the right one. Having a normal conversation or writing books was no longer an option. Afterwards he learned to make use of a computer and a speech system, which were built into his wheelchair. In his autobiography '*My brief history*' Hawking describes his life and career, including his illness. The biographic film '*The theory of everything*' (director John Marsh, 2014) tells the life story of Hawking and is based on the Jane Hawking's book '*Travelling to infinity. My life with Stephen*' (2012). Hawking died on March 14, 2018.

In 1996 Australian Zana Walker was diagnosed with ALS. She was told that she had only another 3 or 4 years to live. But twelve years later she was still alive and she wrote her touching, but often also optimistic life story in her book '*Legless in the garden*'. She tells how she succeeded to survive in spite of all the negativity she experienced from the medical world and how she kept functioning independently in spite of meeting great opposition.

An extraordinary autobiographical book on dysarthria is titled '*In conversation with a speech impediment*' (original Dutch title: 'In gesprek met een spraakgebrek'). The author, Dutch Karen Hekking (°1971) speaks "differently". Different from others and different from before. The special thing is that she once was a speech therapist, but now is suffering from dysarthria herself. She describes her personal quest for a real conversation after having lost her speech. How do you make real contact when speaking is no longer automatic and obvious? Hekking has now 'celebrated' her ten-year anniversary with her speech problem. In her book she states that real communication actually has tremendously little to do with speaking. The ways in which she makes contact, seeks connection, perceives and tries to understand the others have proved many times more important. We quote a short excerpt from the introduction of her remarkable book:

> "Time and again I went wrong. Misunderstanding arose, misunderstandings grew into hassle. That bothered me and my conversation partners. I failed in public. I faced shame, guilt, and fear. Social isolation seemed like an insanely attractive alternative to my verbal fumbling. I couldn't do it to anyone else to have a conversation with me. Loneliness was perhaps not so bad. It suddenly seemed so logical to shut up, now that I had become who I did not wanted to be. I would have conversations again if I could speak "normally" again. But I didn't learn to speak "normally" again. (p. 8).

'*Gaby Brimmer: An autobiography in three voices*' is the life story of Gaby Brimmer (1947-2000). This Mexican woman was the daughter of Austrian Jewish immigrants. Due to rh-incompatibility she showed a severe form of cerebral palsy at birth. At school one of her teachers noticed that she had a well-developed feeling for language and he encouraged her to start writing. She did so using her left foot and a typewriter. In spite of a lot of opposition, she became a writer and an important advocate for the rights of people with disabilities. '*Gaby. A true story*' is the film adaptation of this book, dating from 1987 and starring Liv Ullmann among others.

The autobiography '*My left foot*' by the Irish Christy Brown shows some resemblance to Brimmer's. Brown also only has

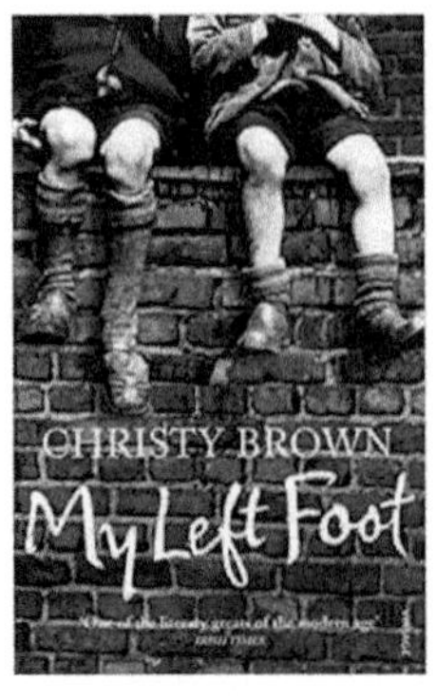

motor control of his left foot to express himself. As a baby and a toddler he couldn't lift his head and neither could he control any of his extremities. A pivotal scene in the book is the moment the boys shows to be intelligent. At the age of five, he grabs a piece of chalk with his foot and writes the letter 'A' on the floor. Later he discovers his creative and artistic gifts and devotes himself to writing and painting. The story of Brown's life has been adapted for the movies in 1989 by Jim Sheridan, starring Daniel Day Lewis, who received an Oscar for this performance.

'*Annie's coming out*' tells the story of Anne McDonald, a non-speaking Australian woman with cerebral palsy and an intellectual impairment. The book focuses on her life at and her discharge from an institution for the disabled, but also on the attempts of her therapist to try to learn her to communicate using the somewhat controversial method of facilitated communication. This biography was also adapted for the screen in 1984.

'*I Raise My Eyes to Say Yes*' by Ruth Sienkiewicz-Mercer and Steven B. Kaplan is in a certain sense comparable to Martin Pistorius' book 'Ghost boy' (see earlier). As a child, Ruth was completely paralyzed due to cerebral palsy, caused by encephalitis at the age of five weeks. From then onwards she is confined to her bed and wheelchair and permanently dependent on help. This autobiographic book is written with the help of a close friend, who taught her to speak with words, characters and gestures through a special reading board. Ruth, at first degraded to an inhuman being, turns out to be a genius, blessed with a rare spirit, which was also her salvation. The book is shocking

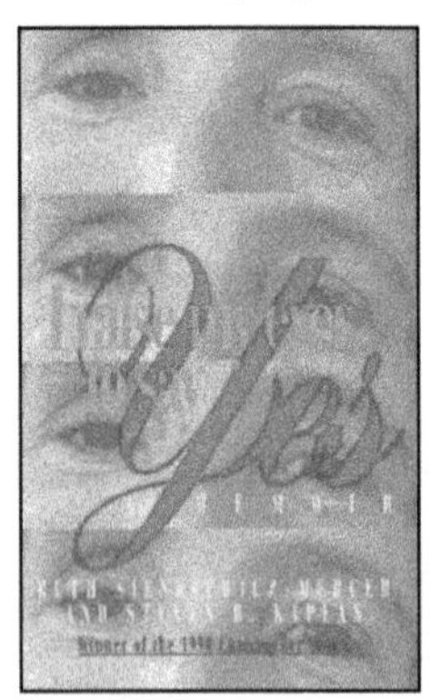

because of her great suffering, especially inflicted by healthcare facilities and caregivers. It's also sort of an indictment of the US health care system. Thanks to her parents and with the help of some good and expert care providers, her treatment and her condition have changed. Ruth now lives with her disabled husband, they try to live with limited financial resources and to spread their message.

Fiction

We 'd like two mention three fiction books, in which characters with dysarthria are the protagonists. By Lisa Genova, who also wrote the captivating novel *'Still Alice'* featuring a woman with young-onset dementia, is the book *'Every note played'*. Richard is a well-respected pianist, who is diagnosed with ALS. The unrelenting progressive symptoms of paralysis occur first of all in his hands, preventing him from playing the piano. He becomes more and more dependent from his surroundings and especially from Katrina, who takes care of him. Finally his muscles, his voice and his respiration all start to cease functioning.

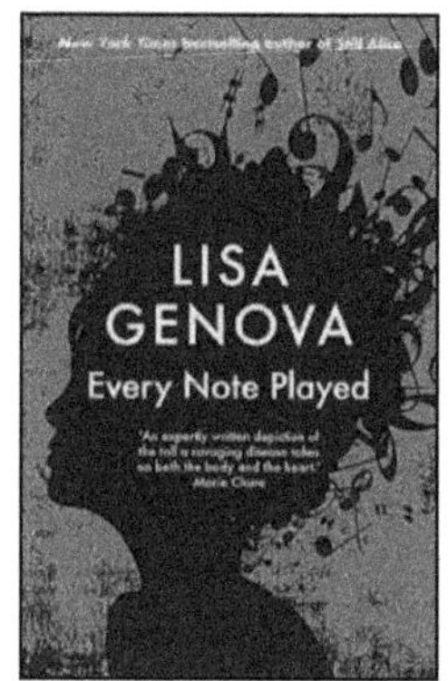

In *'Kayla's dream'* by Theresa Hudson, Kayla is a 22-year old student, who looks forward to a career as a radio presenter. She craves to the moment people will notice Kayla first and not her purple wheelchair or the Dynavox speech device, she uses to communicate. She dreams of Jerome, a handsome and sporty engineering student, but Marc, the director of the radio broadcaster, is secretly in love with her. This story allows the reader to empathize with the experiences and setbacks from the perspective of a young woman with physical limitations and speech difficulties.

A somewhat older but very interesting book, written by William Horwood, is '*Skallagrigg*' (1987). The plot is influenced by the relation between the writer and his daughter Rachel, who suffers from cerebral palsy. It's quite remarkable that Horwood kind of predicted the importance of adapted computer devices to ameliorate the life of future generations of persons with disabilities. The story deals with Arthur, a boy with CP, who is unable to walk, talk, eat independently or even sit without support. His family leaves him in a hospital, thinking that he will be taken care of in the best circumstances. In reality he is confronted with extreme cruelty and negligence, which he tries to escape by making up stories about Skallagrigg, an extraordinary creature with great empathy for the disabled. Many years later Esther, a girl also suffering from CP, becomes interested in Arthur and in Skallagrigg and she starts searching for the history of the treatment of persons with disabilities. A the same time Esther's father brings home a computer and together with a friend she starts programming. They even find a way to use it for facilitating communication.

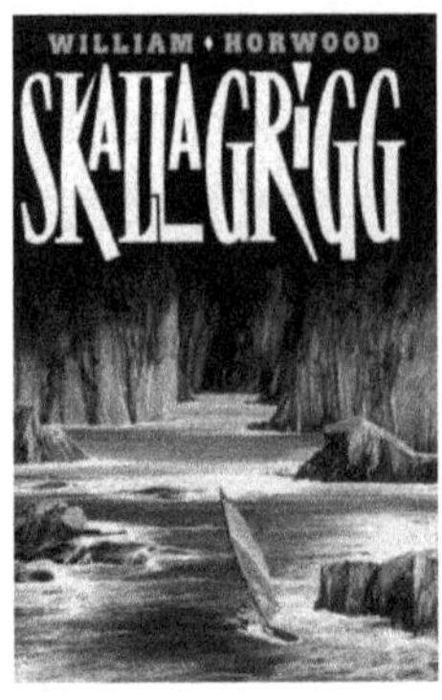

Children's books – young adult

'*Out of my mind*' by Sharon Draper is a **young adult** book about a girl called Melody. She is not like the others, because, due to CP, she can't walk nor talk. On the other hand she has a photographic memory: she can recall every detail of what she has ever experienced. One day she discovers a way to make herself understood. But not everyone in her surroundings seems ready to hear her voice.

Somewhat in the same line is the book *'Stuck in neutral'* by Terry Trueman, intended for young adults from +/- 12 years onward. The narrator of the book is called Shawn McDaniel, a 14-year-old boy with cerebral palsy. His entire body has been affected by the condition and he has no control over his bodily functions. But he also talks about his strengths, such as his perfect memory. Shawn remembers every experience, every sensation, and everything he ever learned in school or saw on television. Unfortunately, due to his lack of motor control, he is unable to talk or make contact with his family members, who therefore assume that he does not have higher functional skills. Shawn indicates several times in the book that he hates to be treated like a baby. Then he gets the impression that his father actually wants him dead. After all, he constantly talks about euthanasia.

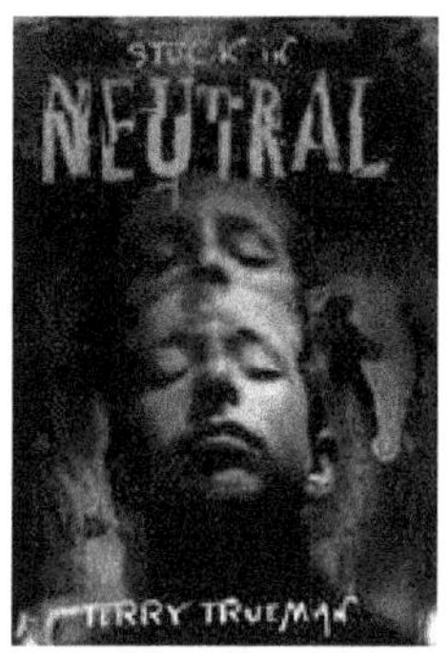

Trueman wrote a sequel to *'Stuck in neutral'*, entitled *'Life happens next'*. Shawn now has a new perspective in his life, but nobody notices. That's because they only see his wheelchair, his paralyzed body, his drooling. They don't notice his brain and his perfect memory, nor his heart beating for a girl he's in love with. How can you connect with someone when you can't talk, can't walk, can't even wave your hand. Things change when his cousin Debi, who suffers from Down syndrome, comes into his life. At first Debi thinks Shawn is very weird and his dog Rusty is even very hostile to him, but after a while the cousin and the dog get a better view of Shawn than anyone else.

We also found some **children's books**, most of them about kids suffering from CP and thus showing dysarthria.

'I'm the Big Sister Now' is an somewhat older book (1989) by Michelle Emmert, intended for children 8 to 10 years old. The nine-year-old Michelle describes the moments of love and joy,

as well as the difficulties and special situations she experienced with her older sister Amy, who was born with very severe disabilities due to cerebral palsy.

Murray Stenton's book is titled *'My Brother Is Special: A Cerebral Palsy Story'*. The author's eldest son suffered a cerebral hemorrhage at birth, which caused cerebral palsy and other complications. The book tells the story of 10-year-old Ethan. He is a big brother like no other. After all, he was born with CP. This poses several challenges, not only for himself, but also for his parents and for his younger brother. The thoughts and feelings of brothers and sisters of children with special needs are also addressed in this book. This book has elicited both positive and negative reviews. Some think that it perpetuates negative stereotypes about people with disabilities, others argue that it helps to shine some light on the difficulties that siblings of special needs children experience every day.

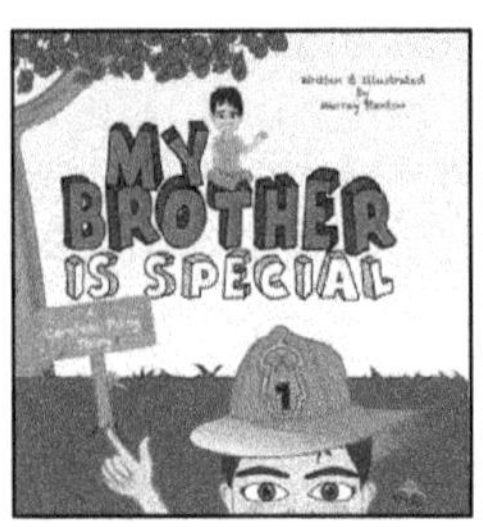

C. Fran Card wrote the booklet *'Ceana has CP'* illustrated by Violet Freeland to help her granddaughter understand what cerebral palsy is. It's a story for children from 3 to +/- 7 years old. In doing so, the author hopes to dispel a number of misconceptions and prejudices that often arise in early childhood.

'Ben's Adventures: Day at the Beach' (2018) and *'Ben's Adventures: Under the Big Top!'* (2019) are two award-winning books, written by Elizabeth Gerlach. The main character is Ben, who cannot walk and cannot talk, but uses his imagination every day. The books are intended for children aged four to eight and can teach all children a lot about empathy, acceptance and friendship. The author was inspired by her own son Benjamin, who suffers from cerebral palsy, when writing.

'The Adventures of Jackpants! is the story of a superhero, Jack Bennion, written and illustrated by his father John. Jack was born four months prematurely and his birthweight was only 1.2 kg. Due to this premature birth, he developed microcephaly and cerebral palsy. These conditions greatly affected his cognition, mobility and speech, but not his zest for life. For children from 4 to 10 years old.

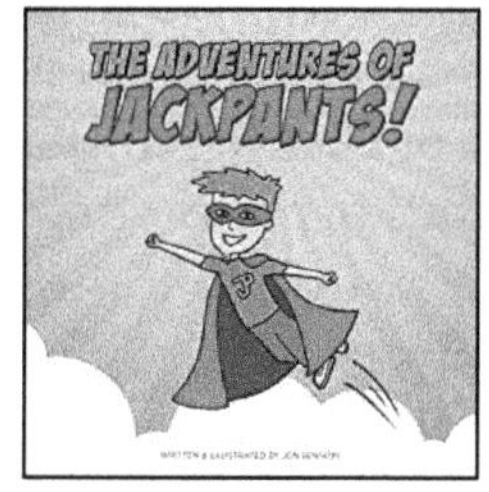

Shaila Abdullah co-wrote *'My Friend Suhana: A Story of Friendship and Cerebral Palsy'* with her daughter Aanyah. When she was seven and her mother was helping in a special education class, Aanyah became friends with Suhanna. The latter could not walk, talk, play, could not answer when called, could not play tag or cycle like other children. But Aanyah helps her in other ways.

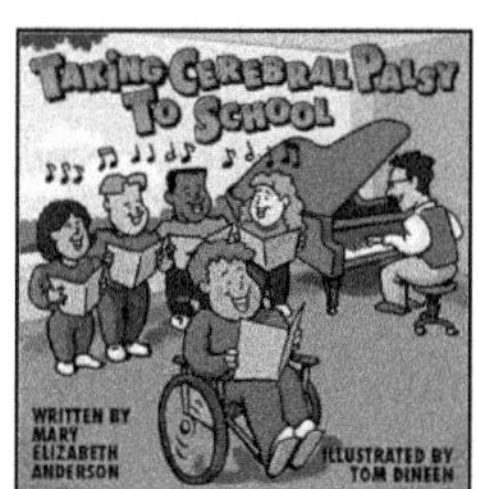

'Taking Cerebral Palsy To School' by M.E. Anderson describes the adventures of Chad, a boy with CP, and his classmates. The book tries to answer the many questions that peers of children with CP may have. This is done in a way that teaches them to empathize and to understand and accept the challenges children with CP experience in the classroom. For ages 5 or older.

Films

Most **films** in which people with motor impairments and dysarthria play a role, are based on true life stories. Some examples are the higher mentioned biographic films featuring Stephen Hawking, Christy Brown and Gaby Brimmer.

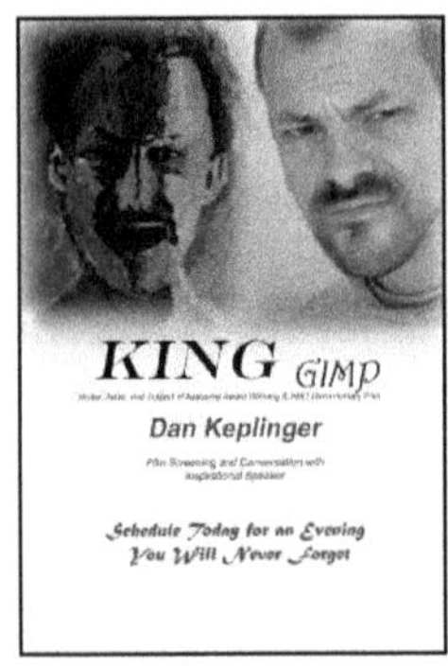

'*King Gimp*' is a non-fiction film from 1999, that has been rewarded with an Oscar for best short documentary film in 2000. It follows the life of Dan Keplinger, who suffers from CP since his birth, from the age of 13. Although not evident, he's attending regular education at that moment. Later on, he graduates, moves from his mother's house to his own apartment and has his first exhibition as a painter. Also today he's mainly busy with painting. His speech is still difficult to understand due to a severe form of dysarthria.

The script of the film '*Dance me to my song*' was written by Heather Rose, who also plays the leading part. Rose (1966-2000) was born with severe CP and was wheelchair bound since childhood. She also had to make use of a speech device to communicate. The film is largely autobiographic. It tells the story of Julia, who is completely dependent from her caretaker Madeleine. The latter is not really nice for Julia, calls her 'spaz', leaves her behind on the toilet and forces her to witness her escapades with several lovers. One day Julia meets Eddie, who becomes her buddy, making Madeleine jealous.

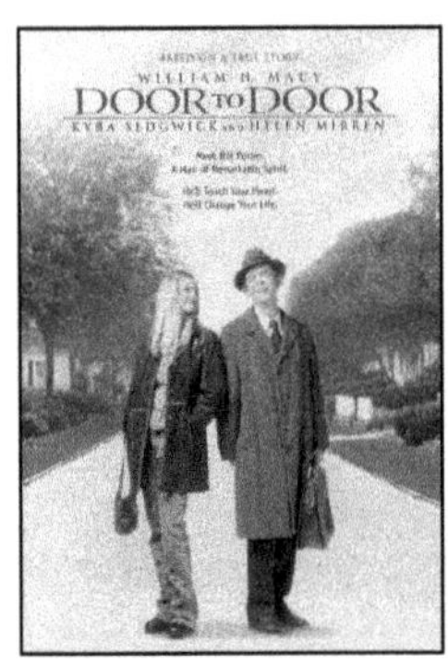

The biographic film '*Door to door*' (2002) is based on the life of Bill Porter, an inspiring and successful door-to-door salesman, also suffering from CP. This touching portrait, directed by Steven Schachter, was nominated for 12 Emmy-awards and won six of those. For years Porter had been told that he was unable to work, but he was determined to succeed and to make it as a salesman. In spite of his clumsiness, his laborious speech and the constant pain he had to endure, he sometimes walked 10 miles a day to meet his clients.

'*Margarita with a straw*' is an Indian film from 2014, produced by Shonali Bose. Laila is a Indian teenager suffering from CP, who receives a grant to study in the US for six months. With her mother, she moves to Greenwich Village. There she meets a nice boy, who helps her with her lessons on creative writing, but she's also introduced to the blind activist Khanum, who she falls in love with. Although Kalki Koechlin, who plays the leading part, doesn't have CP, she plays the role of Laila very lifelike. The title is derived from the fact that Laila has to drink her cocktails with a straw.

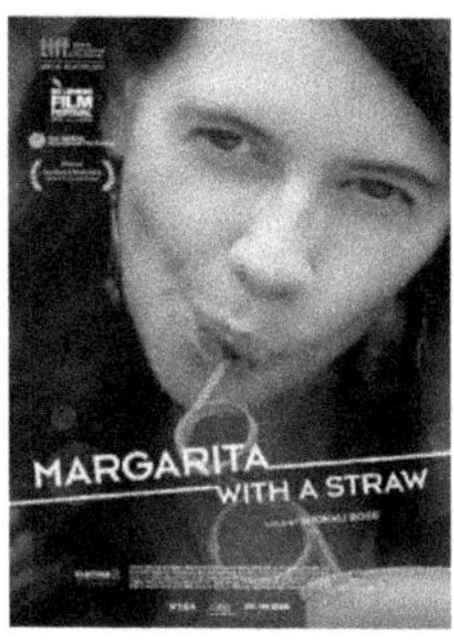

For the sake of completeness we also mention three other Indian movies, featuring persons with CP and dysarthria: '*Tera Mera Saath Rahen*' (2001), '*Vinmeengal*' (2012) and '*Zero*' (2018). The film '*Oasis*' was made in South-Korea and tells the story of a relationship between a boy who shows an intellectual impairment and a girl who has CP.

References chapter 3

Abdullah, S. (2014). *My Friend Suhana: A Story of Friendship and Cerebral Palsy*. Loving Healing Press.

Anderson, E. (2000). *Taking Cerebral Palsy to School*. JayJo Books.

Bennion, J. (2015). *The Adventures of Jackpants*. Alphagrafics (Kindle edition).

Brimmer, G. (2009). *Gaby Brimmer: An Autobiography in Three Voices*. Brandeis University Press, Waltham.

Brown, C. (1954). *My Left Foot*. Collins Educational, London.

Card, C.F. (2006). *Ceanna has CP*. Royal Blue Books

Crossley, R. , McDonald, A. (1985). *Annie's Coming Out*. Penguin Books, London.

Darley, F., Aronson, A., Brown, J. (1975). *Motor Speech Disorders*. Saunders, Philadephia.
Draper, S. (2018). *Out of my mind.* Simon & Schuster, New York.
Emmert, M. (1989). *I'm the Big Sister Now*. Concept Books
Genova, L. (2019). *Every note played*. Allen & Unwin.
Gerlach, E. (2018). *Ben's Adventures: Day at the Beach*. Charley House Press.
Gerlach, E. (2019). *Ben's Adventures: Under the big top!* Charley House Press.
Hawking, J. (2012). *Travelling to infinity. My life with Stephen*. Alma Books, London.
Hawking, S. (2013) *My brief history*. Bantam Press, London.
Hekking, K. (2019). *In gesprek met een spraakgebrek*. Het boekenschap, Zellem.
Horwood, W. (1987). *Skallagrigg*. Penguin books, London.
Hudson, T. (2014). *Kayla's dream*. Xlibris, Bloomington.
Stenton, M. (2016). *My Brother Is Special: A Cerebral Palsy Story*. Loving Healing Press.
Trueman, T. (2012). *Stuck in neutral*. HarperTeen, London.
Trueman, T. (2012). *Life happens next*. HarperTeen, London.

Chapter 4: Stuttering

Stuttering[7] is probably the best-known fluency disorder. The speech of a person who stutters is characterized by interruptions in the flow of speech, in the form of hesitations, interruptions, prolongations and/or repetitions (Conture, 2001). Stuttering was and still is a mystery that has attracted interest for a long time yet. There is still much uncertainty and speculation about the causes and the best treatment.

Examples of people who stutter can be traced back centuries (Brosch & Pirsig, 2001). We think of the Greek Demosthenes, who tried to control his fluency by putting pebbles in his mouth, and of Moses, who is also said to have stuttered. In the Book of Exodus, Moses says to God, "Oh Lord, I have never been a man of fluent speech, never in my life, even though You have spoken to me. My speech is slow and hesitant ".

Another ancient example of a person who stutters (PWS) is the Roman emperor Claudius, about whom Graves wrote a semi-biographical book in 1934, of which later a 13-part television series was made (see below). Other famous persons who stuttered were King George VI of England, about whom the beautiful film *'The King's Speech'* was made (see also below) and Sir Winston Churchill. The latter thought that his slight dysfluencies added an interesting element to his speech. He once stated: "Sometimes a mild and not unpleasant stutter can help to secure the attention of the audience". 'The Stuttering Foundation' has published a list of famous people who stutter or have stuttered, amongst them the actress Marilyn Monroe and the current president of the USA Joe Biden. In popular culture we find many references to persons who stutter (PWS).

---

[7] We have chosen to use 'stuttering', although we are aware of the fact that in the U.K. the term 'stammering' is more prevailing.

Due to the unusual sounding speech, as well as the frequently occurring secondary behaviors (fear of speaking, avoidance behavior, ...) and the attitudes associated with stuttering, this speech disorder has often been the subject of scientific interest and curiosity, but also of discrimination, scorn and mockery.

In this chapter we make a distinction between (1) (auto)biographical and non-fiction books, (2) fiction stories, (3) films, music and theater and (4) children's and youth books. The offer is again overwhelming, forcing us to make a selection.

(Auto)biographies and non-fiction.

'Out with It: How Stuttering Helped Me Find My Voice' is a book by Katherine Preston. The author, who herself started to stutter around the age of seven, tries in this book to shed light on a disorder that affects +/- 60 million people worldwide. She has made an anthology of experiences and expertise. She did speak not only to specialists in the field, but also to famous persons, writers, musicians, social workers, psychologists, people from the financial world. There were both men and women. They all have in common that in the course of their lives they have fought with their speech. What began as a quest for a cure became for Preston a journey to uncover a whole series of misunderstandings about stuttering.

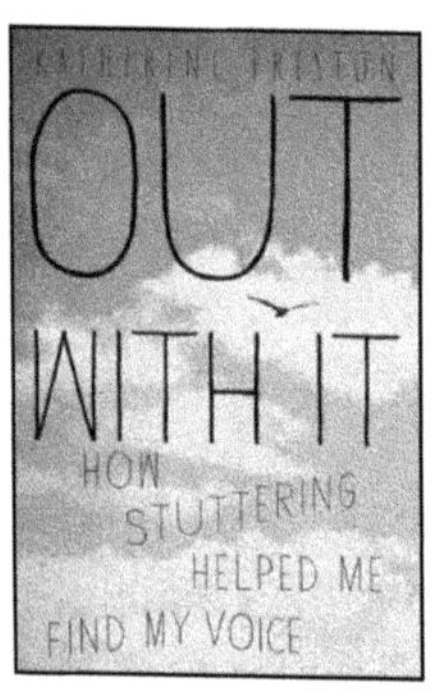

In their investigation on the use of bibliotherapy in which six graduate students in speech-language pathology and five adult clients who stuttered participated, Gerlach and Subramanian (2016) made use of the memoir *'Out with it'*. Book discussions were used as a supplemental therapeutic strategy, and typically lasted for 15–30 min of each session. As a result graduate students reported developing essential clinical skills for working with clients who stutter, including an improved understanding of the experiences of PWS and an increased ability to form and strengthen the therapeutic alliance. Clients reported experiencing shifts in the cognitive and affective components of the disorder. The authors conclude that bibliotherapy can be an effective tool in therapy and clinical education concerning fluency disorders when used appropriately.

'Stuttering: A Life Bound Up in Words' was written by Marty Jezer, a political activist and journalist. He describes how, although stuttering had an impact on his life, it never prevented him from doing what he wanted to do.

In *'Jackdaw Cake. An Autobiography'* Norman Lewis describes changing from a stuttering schoolboy to a worldly-wise, multilingual secret agent and well-known travel author.

'A Stutterer's Story' was written by Frederick P. Murray and published by the Stuttering Foundation of America. It is an autobiography of a person with a severe fluency problem. Although he had reached a fragile degree of fluency a number of times, he also relapsed several times. Murray believes that, regardless of severity, individuals who stutter can reach an acceptable level of fluency and find a workable solution to their difficulties.

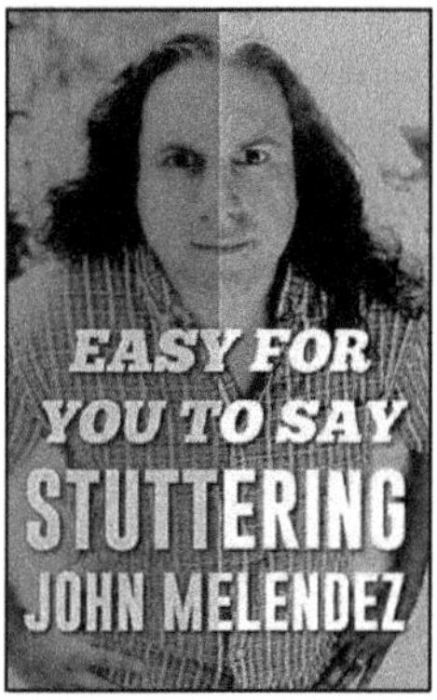

'Easy For You To Say Stuttering' is the autobiography of John Melendez. He describes how he was bullied at school as a child because of his stuttering. Melendez has come to be known as 'Stuttering John'. He is an American radio personality, comedian, actor, writer and more. From 1988 to 2004 he worked on the Howard Stern show, in which he

asked all kinds of impertinent questions to all kinds of celebrities while stuttering.
He later also collaborated on the Tonight Show with Jay Leno. In April 2018 he launched the 'Stuttering John' - Podcast. This and much more is discussed in this book.

Joseph Cooper wrote *'Autobiography of a stutterer'*. In this book he describes the past fifteen years of his life as a stutterer. In this way he wants to give the reader the opportunity to learn from first source what it is like to stutter. By following the instructions to mimic the symptoms of a fluency disorder, the problems with communication and understanding will surface. Although the psychological impact and inhibitions caused by the disorder will of course elude non-stutterers, they will be able to sense somewhat the mechanical aspect of the speech disturbances and the frustrating interruptions themselves.

'Stutterer Interrupted: The Comedian Who Almost Didn't Happen' is a recent book written by Nina G. She describes herself as 'The San Francisco Bay Area's Only Female Stuttering Comedian'. On stage she is occasionally interrupted by someone from the audience, but especially outside of it she is often confronted with comments about her stuttering: people who finish her sentences, ask her if she has forgotten her name or give her unwanted advice such as "Speak a little slower and take a deep breath first". When Nina started as a stand-up comedian ten years ago, she was the first woman in that branch to stutter, which is not surprising since many more men than women stutter and the world of comedy is a man's bastion anyway.

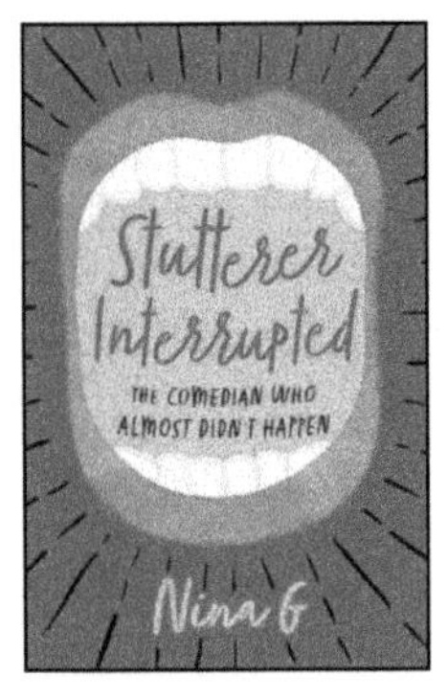

As a stepping stone to the section on fictional stories, we describe below a number of biographical data on famous authors, who themselves had a stuttering problem.

In an interview, the famous American writer John Updike (1932-2009) explains how his stuttering led him to become a writer. "You know," he says, "you write because you can't speak very well, and one of the reasons I was determined to write was because I wasn't an orator like my mother and grandfather were. They were both able to speak beautifully and did so constantly". In his memoirs *'Self-Consciousness,'* he wrote an essay on stuttering entitled *'Getting the Words Out'*, in which he describes his experiences as a stutterer as "... a kind of window glass that was suddenly placed in front of my face while I talked. It was... an insurmountable screen thrown up my throat". Updike states that he still stuttered from time to time as an adult, but that things got better with the years.

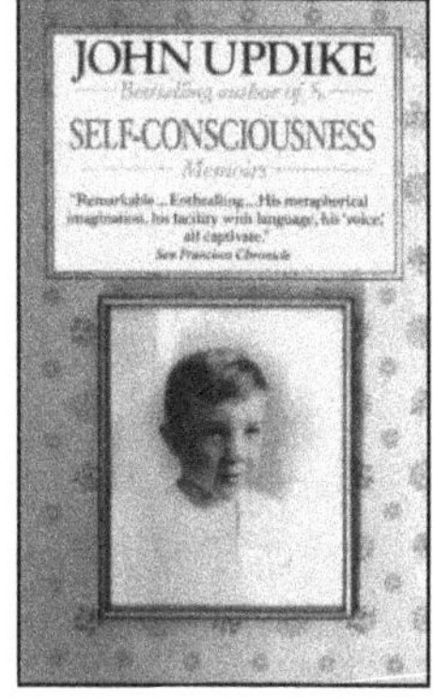

The equally famous British writer William Somerset Maugham has also stuttered his entire life. His childhood years were full of adversity due to his speech problem. The years he spent at 'The King's School' in Canterbury must have been especially hell. In his memoirs recorded by Jeffrey Myers (2005), he says: "When an evil teacher asked me to translate a passage and I started to stutter, the other boys started laughing and the teacher shouted "Sit back, you idiot, I don't know why they put you in this class". Seventy years later, Somerset Maugham still remembered that scornful laughter from his teacher and from his classmates and the humiliation that came with it. One of his best-known works is the semi-autobiographical *'Of human bondage'*, in which the protagonist does not stutter, but is laughed at by his peers because he has a clubfoot. Although stuttering is not mentioned in this book, the experiences and emotions that accompany it are very similar and very present.

Finally we mention Lewis Carroll, the author of *'Alice in Wonderland'*, who had problems with stuttering since childhood and continued to speak dysfluently throughout his life. Although it is claimed that he only stuttered in the company of adults and spoke fluently to children, there is no real evidence of this. It is said that he named the Dodo in "Alice in Wonderland" after his own name. His real name was Dodgson, but he pronounced it Do-Do-Dodgson. In any case, he often referred to himself as "the dodo", possibly referring to his stuttering problem. In his comprehensive overview of Carroll's life, the biographer John Pudney wrote: "Perhaps his failure to correct his speech impediment was the overarching symbol of his entire life. He learned to live with his stammering; he knew what it permitted him to do, what not, where it would snare him and destroy the effects he sought to achieve and how to avoid the traps." Carroll undertook speech therapy lessons from James Hunt, who was considered the foremost speech correctionist in Great Britain at the time (Stuttering Foundation Magazine, 2020).

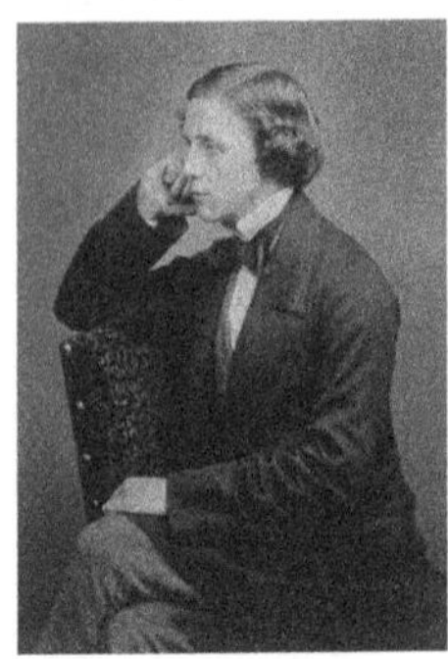

In *'Alice in Wonderland'* multiple instances can be found of advices Carroll may have got about his stuttering from the people with whom he spoke. Several striking examples are found in the dialogue between Alice and the Red Queen:

> *"'It's time for you to answer now,' the Queen said, looking at her watch, 'Open your mouth a little wider when you speak...'"*

> *"Look up, speak nicely, and don't twiddle your fingers"*
> *"Think before you speak. Write it down afterward!"*

Fiction

In a short article from 1976, Trotter and Silverman list 27 novels, biographies, short stories and plays featuring persons who stutter (PWS). Many years later an update appeared, with a number of additions of more recent date (Kuster, 2008). The authors indicate that such a list can be of interest to speech therapists for several reasons. Firstly, the picture sketched in the literature of PWS reflects and influences the impression that exists of them in real society. Moreover, such works can be used in therapy as a starting point and in facilitating discussions about the attitude towards one's own stuttering. For example, one could ask an PWS to read some works and then discuss his/her reactions to how stutterers are represented with the therapist. Trotter and Silverman argue that PWS are certainly not depicted in a stereotypical way in these books. They fulfill, just to name one thing, very different roles, such as that of detective ('Petrovka 38' by Julian Semyonov, 1965), of football coach ('Two hours on Sunday', Pillitteri, 1971), of psychopathic nymphomaniac ('The quick red fox' by McDonald, 1964) and of participant in a hostage situation ('The revolution script', Moore, 1971).

Just as in films (see below), in literature stuttering behavior all too often serves a comic function. Stuttering is then characterized by highlighting the laughable features of the disorder (Cabrera, 2001). If the PWS ends up in a predicament (speaking) situation, this arouses laughter, just as is the case when someone sees someone else stumble or when someone is dressed inappropriately. In addition, characters who stutter are often portrayed in books as pitiable or as not fully social and/or emotional. They are seldom presented as strong and healthy personalities, which is of course unfortunate and unjustified. We give a number of examples of PWS, which are presented in novels.

In the first chapter of Gustave Flaubert's debut novel *'Madame Bovary'* from 1856, Charles Bovary enters his new class for the first time. The following situation takes place, a striking example of a PWS, who is laughed at, as described above. We cite a fragment:

> "Rise," said the master.

He stood up; his cap fell. The whole class began to laugh. He stooped to pick it up. A neighbour knocked it down again with his elbow; he picked it up once more.

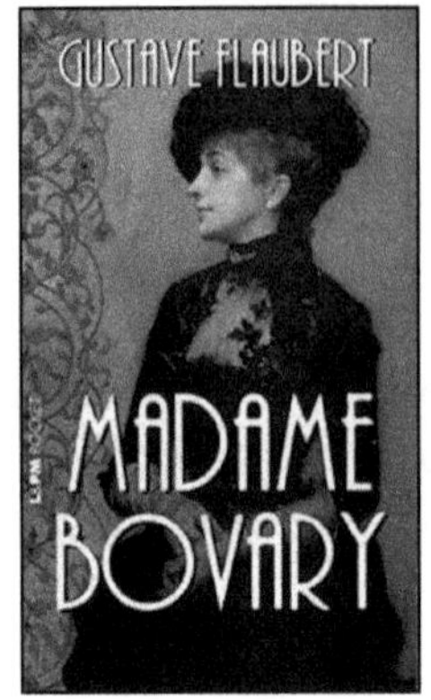

"Get rid of your helmet," said the master, who was a bit of a wag.

There was a burst of laughter from the boys, which so thoroughly put the poor lad out of countenance that he did not know whether to keep his cap in his hand, leave it on the ground, or put it on his head. He sat down again and placed it on his knee.

"Rise," repeated the master, "and tell me your name."

The new boy articulated in a stammering voice an unintelligible name.

"Again!"

The same sputtering of syllables was heard, drowned by the tittering of the class.

"Louder!" cried the master; "louder!"

The "new fellow" then took a supreme resolution, opened an inordinately large mouth, and shouted at the top of his voice as if calling someone in the word "Charbovari."

A hubbub broke out, rose in crescendo with bursts of shrill voices (they yelled, barked, stamped, repeated "Charbovari! Charbovari"),....

Nosy Barbon is the stuttering admirer of painter Guley Jimson in Joyce Cary's 1944 Book *'The Horse's Mouth'*. The book was later, in 1958, also made into a film.

The novel *'Brideshead Revisited'*, written by Evelyn Waugh in 1945 and later adapted for the screen, features a certain

Anthony Blanche. This one is the gay friend of the Brideshead estate's son of the house and an intellectual and esthete, whose keen humor and shrewd criticism impress his fellow Oxford students. The main character describes his first encounter with this Blanche in the following way:

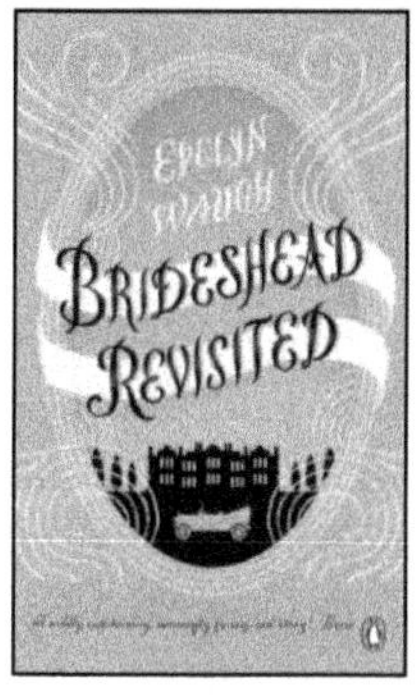

'When the eggs were gone and we were eating the lobster Newburg, the last guest arrived .'My dear,' he said, 'I couldn't get away before. I was lunching with my p-p-preposterous tutor. He thought it was very odd my leaving when I did. I told him I had to change for F-f-footer. .....

This, I did not need telling, was Anthony Blanche, the 'aesthete' par excellence, a byword of iniquity from Cherwell Edge to Somerville. He had been pointed out to me often in the streets, as he pranced along with his high peacock tread; I had heard his voice in the George challenging the conventions; and now meeting him, under the spell of Sebastian, I found myself enjoying him voraciously. After luncheon he stood on the balcony with a megaphone which had appeared surprisingly among the bric-a-brac of Sebastian's room, and in languishing tones recited passages from 'The Waste Land' to the sweatered and muffled throng that was on its way to the river.

'*I, Tiresias, have fore suffered all,*' he sobbed to them from the Venetian arches. '*Enacted on this same d-divan or b-bed ,*
I who have sat by Thebes below the wall
And walked among the l-l-lowest of the dead...'
And then, stepping lightly into the room, 'How I have surprised them! All b-boatmen are Grace Darlings to me.' (p. 21-22)

In the essay '*Stuttering Joyce*' (2011) David Spurr argues that stuttering and other forms of breakdown in the smooth flow of speech occur in James Joyce's work at crucial moments, notably at moments of confession under the pressure of interrogation. He shows how Joyce uses stuttering and other "errors" in correct pronunciation to develop a new literary language that finds its fully achieved form in '*Finnegans Wake*'. We borrow two citations from Spurr's essay, one concerning '*Ulysses*' and the other about '*Finnegans Wake*':

> Deep within the psychic labyrinth of the Circe-episode of '*Ulysses*', the sadistic man-woman Bello demands a singular confession from the protagonist Leopold Bloom: "Say! What is the most revolting piece of obscenity in all your career of crime? Go the whole hog. Puke it out! Be candid for once". Bloom equivocates for a few moments before gurgling docilely: "I rererepugnosed in rerererepugnant...". Under the pressure of violent interrogation, Bloom can only stutter. Even though his answer remains incoherent, one can suppose it inspired by the memory of what is, at least in his own eyes, an act of abjection (Spurr, 2011, p. 121).
>
> A recurring figure from the written word in '*Finnegans Wake*' presents the letter as litter, as in the 'Shem the Penman' chapter, where words ooze and spill out in the form of "burst loveletters [...] alphabettyformed verbiage [...] imeffible tries at speech unasyllabled, etc. The spoken equivalent for the letter as litter is stutter as clutter, inasmuch as speech overflows the limits of standard pronunciation by producing an excess of syllables per word. The stutter is thus a form of vocal noise (Spurr, 2011, p. 127).

In the semi-autobiographical novel '*Black Swan Green*' David Mitchell describes his own experiences as a 13-year-old stutterer.

For example, in the chapter "Hangman" he notes down how the main character, Jason, ends up with the speech therapist after a negative experience in class. We quote an excerpt from the book:

> Miss Throckmorton 'd been playing Hangman on the blackboard one afternoon with sunlight streaming in. On the blackboard was
>
> NIGH–ING––E
>
> Any duh-brain could work that out, so I put up my hand. Miss Throckmorton said, "Yes, Jason?" and that was when my life divided itself into Before Hangman and After Hangman. The word "nightingale" kaboomed in my skull but it just *wouldn't come out*. The 'n' got out okay, but the harder I forced the rest, the tighter the noose got. I remember Lucy Sneads whispering to Angela Bullock, stifling giggles. I remember Robin South staring at this bizarre sight. I'd 've done the same if it hadn't been me. When a stammerer stammers their eyeballs pop out, they go trembly-red like an evenly matched arm wrestler, and their mouth gupperguppergupper like a fish in a net. It must be quite a funny sight. It wasn't funny for me, though. Miss Throckmorton was waiting. Every kid in the classroom was waiting. Every crow and every spider in Black Swan Green was waiting. Every cloud, every car on every motorway, even Mrs. Thatcher in the House of Commons 'd frozen, listening, watching, thinking, *What's* wrong *with Jason Taylor*? But no matter how shocked, scared, breathless, ashamed I was, no matter how much of a total flid I looked, no matter how much I hated myself for not being able to say a simple word in my own language, *I couldn't* say "nightingale." In the

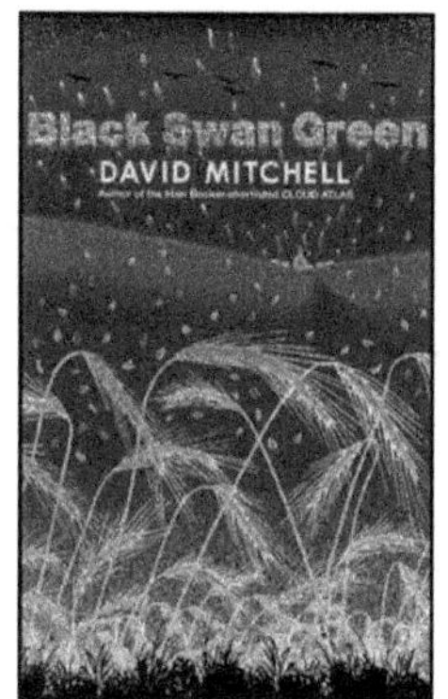

end I had to say, “I’m not sure, miss,” and Miss Throckmorton said, “I see.” She did see, too. She phoned my mum that evening and one week later I was taken to see Mrs. de Roo, the speech therapist at Malvern Link Clinic. That was five years ago. (p. 25).

David Mitchell writes in a contribution to ‘Prospect Magazine’ (2011) that he might still avoid the topic of stuttering if he had not come out as a stutterer through this book. He mentions that until then the topic had been consistently avoided, both in his family and by friends and colleagues on the basis of the reasoning "the poor man must suffer enough without us bringing up the topic." In the same article, the writer is very enthusiastic about the way in which the problem of stuttering is approached in the film *'The King's speech'* (see below) and is very candid about his own speech problems, the misunderstandings that exist about stuttering and the bag of tricks he uses himself to overcome or avoid dysfluencies.

'I, Claudius' is the fictional autobiography of Emperor Clau-Clau-Claudius (10 BC - 54 AD), written by Robert Graves in 1934. Claudius is described as a pitiful stutterer who was destined to become emperor despite himself. Robert Graves describes the eternal intrigue, corruption, bloodshed and increasing cruelty during the reigns of Augustus and Tiberius, which eventually culminated in the deified madness of Caligula, the predecessor of Claudius. The book was turned into a thirteen-part television series by the BBC in 1976. The series, written by Jack Pulman, is based on the books *‘I, Claudius’* and the sequel *‘Claudius, the God’* by Graves. The series meant a breakthrough for various beginning actors such as Derek Jacobi (as the stuttering Claudius), John Hurt (as Caligula) and Patrick Stewart (as Sejanus).

‘Billy Budd’ was the last book written by Herman Melville, best known for *‘Moby Dick’*. It was published posthumously in 1924. The book was later also adapted for theater and opera (in 1951). Later, in 1962, the book was also made into a film (see below).

We briefly outline the story. Billy, a foundling from Bristol, is an innocent-looking, handsome young man. His natural flair makes him much beloved by the ship's crew. His only problem is his stuttering, which gets worse with intense emotion. He provokes the enmity of Petty Officer Claggart, who is jealous of Billy because of his popularity. This leads Claggart to accuse him of complicity in mutiny. When Captain Vere hears about these accusations, he summons both men to his cabin for a meeting. Claggart makes his point, but Billy is taken aback and unable to answer due to his stuttering. The captain, unaware of Billy's speech problem, admonishes him to answer: "Speak, defend yourself!" However, this only has a counterproductive effect. The more he tries to speak, the less he succeeds. Follows a complete blockage of the speech organs, producing not even a stutter, but only "a strange dumb gesturing and gurgling...intensifying it into a convulsed tongue-tie" (p. 98). Extremely frustrated, he lashes out at Claggart, who is killed instantly. Vere convenes an ad hoc court-martial and although everyone is convinced that Claggart has wrongly accused Budd, he is sentenced to death by hanging under the prevailing laws of war. Harison (2011) describes that Billy's "susceptibility to blocking his speech" may be triggered by malicious injustice, here in the person of Claggart. Melville describes stuttering as a dormant, latent defect, as an expression of dismay that wells up from a person who has a hard time forming his words and therefore sees only one way out for justice to prevail, namely by dealing a punch. We will also see this same phenomenon further down in the description of the stuttering boxing champion Rubin "Hurricane" Carter (see films).

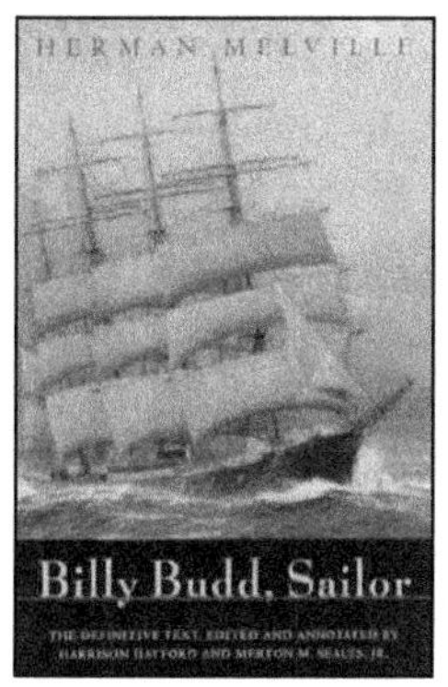

The 1989 book *'Dead languages'* by David Shields is a coming of age novel about a certain Jeremy Zorn. The story is mainly devoted to the protagonist's attempts during puberty and adolescence to overcome his stuttering problem: he remains silent for a long time, starts singing in a chorus, plays a part in the play Othello and even simulates a suicide attempt. What all these coping behaviors have in common is that they end in deep humiliation with stuttering as the main cause over and over again (Müller, 2012). The novel describes the starting point of the stutter, when Jeremy's mother makes him aware of his dysfunction at the age of 4, until the death of the mother, revealing a total lack of communication within the family. This book also contains a lot of autobiographical elements, since Shields himself has a stuttering problem.

One of the characters from Kesey's book '*One flew over the cuckoo's nest*' (and also from the subsequent film) is a person who stutters, namely Billy Bibbitt. In Billy's case, the stuttering occurs at times of nervousness and shame, and the problem gets worse when he is aware of it or when he is being intimidated. The stuttering behavior culminates in the confrontation with the head nurse, who threatens to inform his mother about his sexual exploits. He reacts by saying, "Duh-duh-don't t-tell, M-M-M-Miss Ratched. Duh-Duh-Duh- ". A little later in the story, Bibbit will take his own life. Eagle (2014) speculates that Billy's stutter actually stems from an unresolved Oedipus complex. When asked at some point to try to remember what word he first stuttered on, he says, "Fir-first stutter? First stutter? The first word I said I stuttered: m-m-m-mama ".

In '*All the Kings Men or the Downfall of Willie Stark*' by Robert Penn Warren (1946, revised 1974), Sugar-Boy is the PWS. On page 11 we read:

> And Sugar-Boy's head would twitch, the way it always did when the words were piling up inside of him and couldn't get out, and then he'd start,
> "The b-b-b-b-b— " he would manage to get out and the saliva would spray from his lips like Flit from a Flit gun.

> "The b-b-b-b-bas-tud— he seen me c-c-c— " and here he'd spray the inside of the windshield—"c-c-com-ing." Sugar-Boy couldn't talk, but he could express himself when he got his foot on the accelerator. He wouldn't win any debating contests in high school, but then nobody would ever want to debate with Sugar-Boy.

This book by Warren was adapted for film twice, with great success in 1949, with much less success in 2006.

The novel *'The Temple of the Golden Pavilion'* by Yukio Mishima (1956) is based on true facts. In 1950, the Buddhist priest Hayashi Yoken sets fire to the Golden Temple in Kyoto. This priest is said to have stuttered from childhood, an element that Mishima transposed to his own main character. The story of Mishima takes place in full time of war, before and after the atomic bombs on Nagasaki and Hiroshima. Mizoguchi, a stuttering teenager, is apprenticed to a monastery in Kyoto as a monk. There he falls under the spell of the Golden Pavilion, an ancient temple. For Mizoguchi, that temple represents absolute beauty, the ideal from which he is excluded by his own ugliness and maladjustment. The beauty of the Golden Pavilion prevents him from living and makes him powerless. If the bombs also fail to destroy that beauty, Mizoguchi is forced to take action himself. The Pavilion will be destroyed in a sea of flames and Mizoguchi wants to go down with it. In this way he hopes, in a fierce apotheosis, to be united with the unattainable beauty.

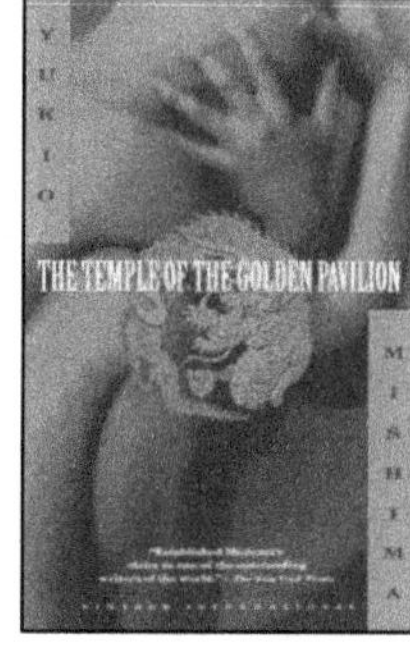

We also mention the recent novel *'Der Stotterer'* (The Stutterer), written by the acclaimed Swiss author Charles Lewinsky, known from his bestseller *'Melnitz'*. It's a book about the power of language, both philosophical and playful. The main character is a person who stutters and therefore trusts entirely in the power of the written word and uses it ruthlessly,

in self-defence and for his career. A fraud case – he calls it a writerly carelessness – has put him in prison. Using letters, avowals and invented stories, he tries to win over the people who have a say over his life behind bars. A quite remarkable book!
We cite a little fragment from the opening:

> With my stutter I made myself interesting to you. You must nurture your talents. I really stutter. In fact, quite bad. And nobody can change that. Stuttering, also called *ballbuties*, is a way of speaking that ...
> Well, just look on the internet. Search term: clonic stuttering.
> (p. 10-11)

In Stephen King's horror story *'It'*, one of the protagonists, Bill, is a member of the so-called Losers Club. The evil spirit 'It', who sometimes appears as the clown Pennywise, makes victims in the town of Derry, including Bill's younger brother. Bill is often referred to as "Stuttering Bill" because of his fluency problems. Although he has a rich vocabulary and is a talented writer, it is very difficult for him to get his words out throughout his childhood. In his teens, Bill overcomes his speech problem by taking speech therapy. Twenty-seven years after the first facts, he is told that "It" has struck again in Derry. He is asked to return, along with the other members of the Losers Club, to fight the evil monster. Bill, in particular, is out to defeat the demon in order to get revenge for what happened to his little brother. At that point, however, the stuttering reappears, especially when he is excited, angry, or anxious. His speech problem is not noticeable when reading in a foreign language, when imitating someone or even when giving a speech. In 1990 the book was

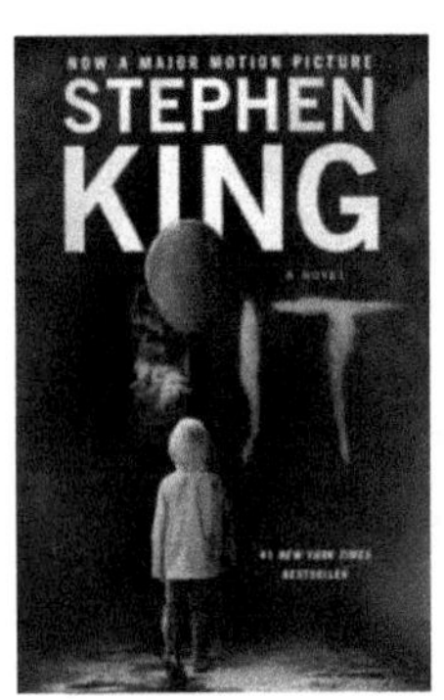

made a two-part miniseries for television, in 2017 the first part of the book was adapted into a full-length film, directed by Andy Muschietti. Here too, 'Stuttering Bill' is one of the main characters.

We came across two novels, in which female characters who stutter are described. In Philip Roth's book *'American Pastoral'* (1997) and Gail Jones' 2007 novel *'Sorry'*, the female protagonists are portrayed as being prone to violent, destructive behavior. Yet the stuttering behavior manifests itself in both girls in an opposite direction. Merry, from Roth's book, develops her stuttering behavior gradually over the course of her childhood, while in Perdita, in Jones's book, it is provoked by the trauma of her father's murder. Yet both stories share the same tendency to link the blocking of speech to sudden outbursts of violence.

'American Pastoral' is about the misery of a man who caused his own misfortune (Buwalda, 1999). The main character is Seymour Levov, who seems to have everything to be happy. He is in love with his homeland, dutiful, hardworking, honest, he feels healthy and happy, marries a nice, beautiful woman and takes over the family business from his father. The only thing 'Dawnie' and he still miss is a child, but there will be. Meredith 'Merry' Levov is born in the early 1950s. For the first eleven years of her life she is a sweet girl who wants to please everyone, her father most of all and she loves the things sweet girls love. There is only one problem: the girl stutters to get scared. Seymour and his wife drag their daughter past speech therapists and psychiatrists for years, who have her keep stuttering diaries and teach her speaking strategies - all to no avail. Merry plunges into puberty, stammering. And then the metamorphosis sets in, so that almost overnight, she grows stout, a bulky, long-strung, dowdy sixteen-year-old nearly six

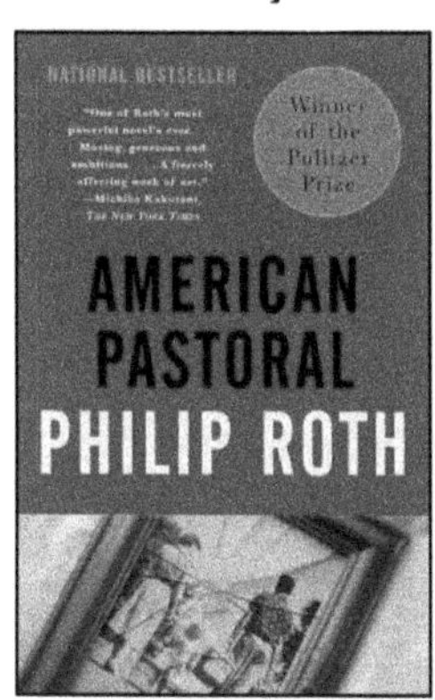

feet tall, nicknamed Ho Chji Levov by her schoolmates. Her stutter becomes the artillery fire she targets at America and the Vietnam War and at every capitalist shitty c-c-c-collaborator helping North Vietnam into its abyss, from President Lyndon B. Johnson himself to "dull cowards" like her parents. Eventually she blows up the Old Rimrock post office and kills the town's family doctor, who just came to post a letter. With one blow, Merry, the happy little daughter Seymour loved to daydream on a swing under the foliage of their apple tree, is forever transformed into the "Rimrock Terrorist." From that moment on, she is wanted by the FBI and goes into hiding. Only five years after the bombing, the father sees his daughter again. Merry is barely recognizable, severely malnourished and dressed in rags. It turns out she has converted to a bizarre, altruistic Indian sect. The child lives in a filthy, dimly lit room in a looted, smelly and desolate Newark neighborhood and sleeps on a narrow foam mattress. She confesses to her father that she blew up not one, but four people. This book was made into a film in 2016, directed by Ewan McGregor, who also plays the lead role himself.

'Sorry' by Gail Jones has Perdita as the main character. The book is set in a tumultuous period of Australian history in the 1940s. Perdita is the daughter of English ex-pats, who are only concerned with themselves and little caring for their daughter. She befriends her neighbor Billy, who is deaf-and-dumb, and Mary, an Aboriginal girl who is brought over by her parents from a monastery to care for Perdita while her mother is in the hospital with a depressed mood. One day, when she returns from a visit to Billy, she witnesses her father raping Mary.

Perdita responds by stabbing her father with a kitchen knife. To protect Perdita, Mary admits to having committed the crime. After these events, the girl appears not only to have developed a (selective) amnesia (she seems to have erased her responsibility for the death of her father), but also a stuttering problem. In the book she herself describes the rarity of her condition as follows:

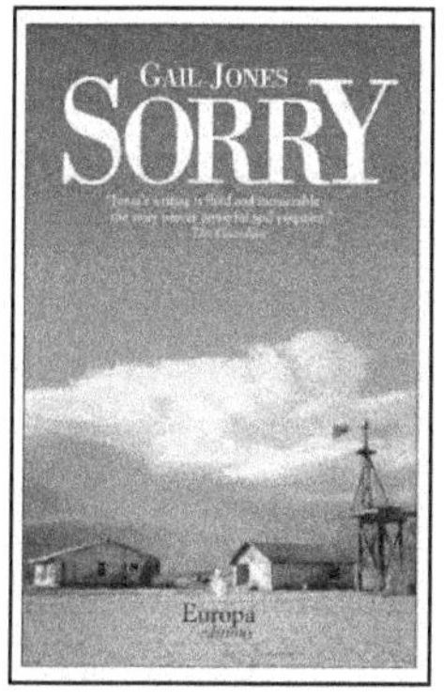

"Of all the anguishing forms of stuttering that can torment children (mostly males, statistically, at least), mine was one of the rarer. Called psychogenic, it is the consequence of shock, or upset or a circumstantial disaster. It is infrequent in its appearance and enigmatic in its cure. Most stuttering is developmental and fades over time; the eruption of stuttering, as it were, is a stranger thing. " (p. 151)

Eventually, Perdita internalizes her stuttering and lapses into such extreme silence that she almost completely loses her voice (Eagle, 2014).

Children's books – young adult

In an article from 1988, Bushey and Martin give an overview of 20 children's books in which a character stutters. In addition to making this overview, which is of course no longer up-to-date, they also examined how the authors of those children's books portray certain aspects of stuttering behavior, such as the symptomatology, the causes and the treatment. This can give us a picture of how stuttering and PWS were presented at the time. After all, as the authors themselves indicate, fiction literature can be used as a means to directly or indirectly influence the thoughts, emotions and attitudes of the reader and thus might have a therapeutic effect. Books provide new ideas and insights about the world, including the internal, psychological and external physical world as well as the complex interpersonal world. A particularly effective clinical and therapeutic application of literature is its use for changing attitudes. Bushey and Martin quote in this regard from an article by Baskin and Harris (1984, p. 30):

> Purely informational books ... have only a modest influence on attitude formation. Novels, however, exhibiting both cognitive and affective appeal, can translate objectively defined societal problems into subjectively realized experiences, creating characters with whom readers can identify, whose emotions they can vicariously share, whose behavior they can imitate, and whose perceptions and judgments they can embrace or reject.

Even today, many stuttering children may benefit from being confronted through stories with characters from books who exhibit a fluency problem. Logan, Mullins and Jones (2008) made a similar overview of children's and youth literature. They reviewed 29 books to find out how the stutter-related content was presented in them. Although the plots and storylines vary widely, many of the characters described exhibit attributes or achievements that counterbalance their communication problem. Many of them make progress in terms of their social and/or communicative functioning, which in some cases happens in combination with professional help. Most books also describe listeners' responses to stuttering, such as impatience, teasing, ridiculing and bullying. Although some books contain misinformation, such as the statement that stuttering is nothing but a symptom of emotional poverty, the images sketched of stuttering are generally more than nuanced enough to be used, among other things, as a means of instruction for pedagogical and therapeutic activities. In the US, the application of so-called bibliotherapy is very common. This means "guiding a person in solving his personal problems through directed reading". This can be done through self-help books as well as fictional stories. There are reasons to argue that fiction stories have the potential not only to influence the reader's thoughts, emotions and attitudes towards particular challenges, but also to impart new and fresh ideas and insights on how best to respond to or deal with problems. Finally, books can also serve to help readers understand that others have experienced and have often overcome problems similar to theirs. As mentioned, Logan, Mullins and Jones took a closer look at 29 children's and youth books that were available and met a number of criteria. It would take us too far to discuss all of these books here (for the full listing, see the article by Logan et al). Suffice it to say that most of the stories (23 out of 29) were set in contemporary settings, which allowed their authors to explore modern views on stuttering without being anachronistic. Of course the stories differed greatly in length, detail and complexity. Some authors are speech therapists or people who stutter themselves. Some books include a foreword or afterword with an explanation of stuttering, written by a speech therapist. In what follows, we include a limited selection of children's and youth books, where stuttering or a PWS is described. Again, we make no effort to strive for completeness. Where we found the information, we always also state for which age(s) the book is intended. There are also some non-fiction books included.

'Sometimes I Just Stutter' (1999) is a book written by the Dutch therapist Eelco de Geus. It has been published by the Stuttering Foundation of America and has been described as a wonderful book for kids of all ages. We cite some of the topics that are dealt with from the table of contents: 'Stuttering is no joke; Sometimes you stutter and sometimes you don't; What makes you stutter; ....; When you get teased about your stuttering; ...; It is alright to stutter!; Tell your own story; Who can help you?; Where to get information'.

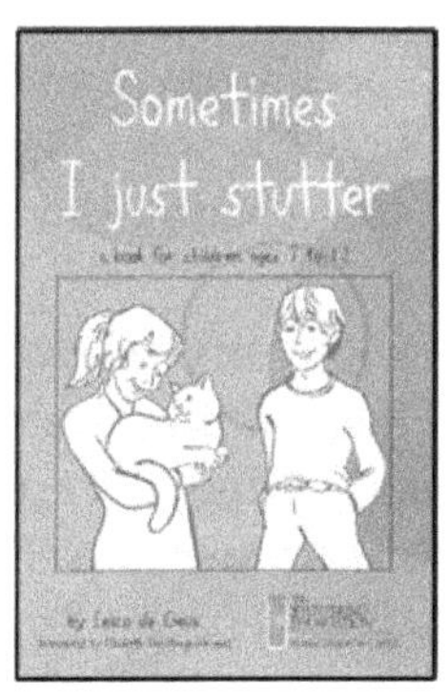

It also contains some letters with advice for brothers and sisters, fathers and mothers, teachers, grandfathers and grandmothers and even for uncles and aunts. A remarkable book!

Kim Block is a PWS herself. She has been an active advocate in the stuttering community for almost twenty years by publishing articles about stuttering, facilitating support groups, and presenting workshops and lectures across Canada and the US. She wrote a series of four children's books, with the title *'Adventures of a Stuttering Superhero'.* These stories talk about stuttering in a way to enhance empathy and acceptance for children who stutter.

The first book has the subtitle *'Interupt-itis'*, the second one *'Melissa Meets her Stamily'*, the third *'Eye contact'* and the fourth is called *'Melissa stays home'*. The first book has also been translated into French (*'Les aventures d'une superhéroine du bégaiement. L'interromptite'*). In addition there's also drawing book *'Why do I stutter? Stuttering adventures. A drawing book'*.

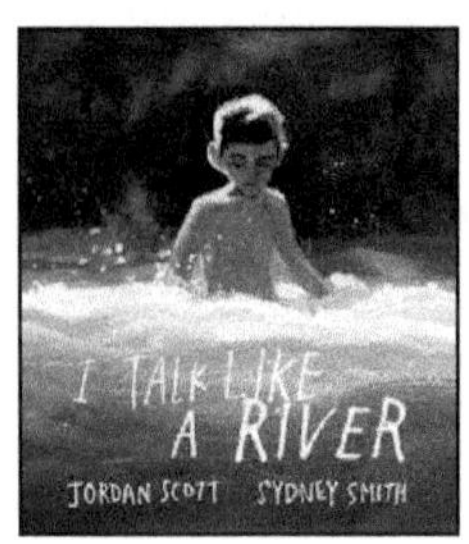

'I Talk Like a River' by Jordan Scott (2020), one of the *New York Times* Best Children's Books of the Year, is based on the writer's own experiences. It is beautifully illustrated by Sydney Smith.
The narrator, a little boy who stutters, sits alone at the kitchen table before school, imagining how badly his day will go. His understanding father knows about a "bad speech day," and takes his son to the river. There he explains how his son talks like the river, with ebbs and flows, a rush of sounds, emotion, and meaning streaming.
When the boy returns to school, he talks about his special place in his own manner, his dysfluency making him and his telling unique. The author Jordan Scott has added a very personal and expressive note to outline the journey he himself has undertaken to make peace with himself.
It's the combination of the breathtaking illustrations and the lyrical text that make this book outstanding. For children 4 to 8 years old.

Scott's story reminded me in a certain sense of the way the renowned Charles Van Riper (1972) depicted stuttering in his book *'Speech Correction'* (see figure below). He also made the comparison between dysfluent speech and the course of a river to explain how stuttering originated and developed.

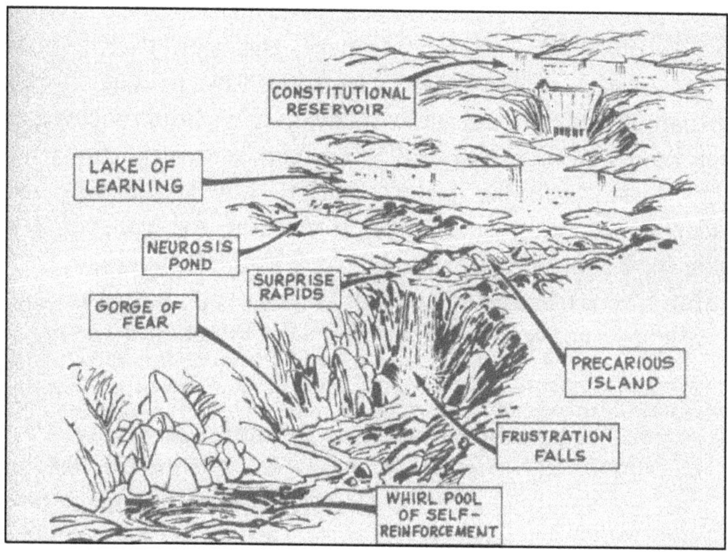

The origin and the development of stuttering according to Charles Van Riper (1972)

'A boy and a jaguar' is an autobiographical story written by Alan Rabinowitz. The author describes the alienation he felt as a child, because he thought that something was broken about him because he could not speak fluently. But he learned there were other, stronger ways to communicate, which he inferred from the ease with which he could talk to animals. As he gets older he learns to deal with the fact that he will always be a person who stutters. He quickly becomes an wildlife conservationist and an advocate for people who stutter. For children from 6 to 10 years old.

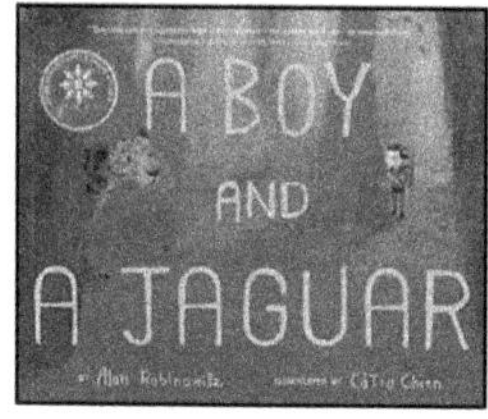

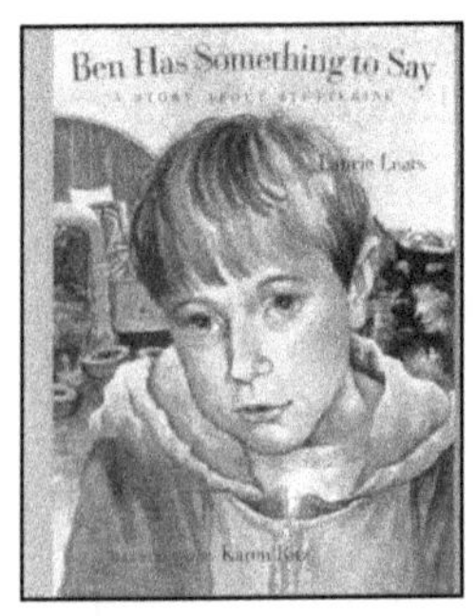

Laurie Lears wrote *'Ben has something to say'*, a book illustrated by Karen Ritz. Ben goes to a junkyard with his father every Friday, looking for parts. There the boy befriends the guard dog. He tries to make it clear to the owner that he should take better care of the dog, but he doesn't succeed because of his stuttering. When, after a burglary, the man threatens to dispose of the dog for being too friendly to guard, Ben eventually finds the courage to ask him if he can buy the dog. When he goes home with Spike, he has discovered that what he has to say is more important than how he says it. The booklet also contains useful information for parents and teachers. It's an inspirational story, that is invaluable for children who stutter or for the people from their surroundings. For children aged 5 and over.

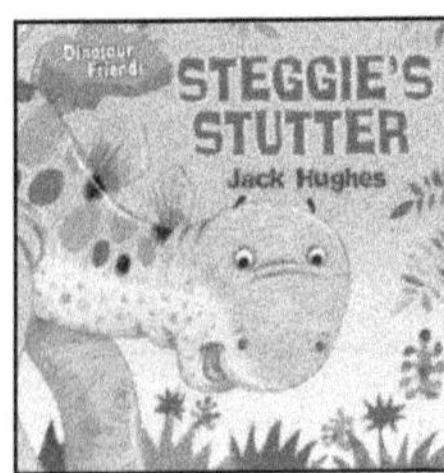

In Jack Hughes' *'Steggie's Stutter'*, Steggie the dinosaur is the one who stutters. He sometimes needs some time to get his words out. His friends are in a rush to play and run away quickly, disregarding Steggie's warnings not to play in the great, dark and eerie forest. Steggie wants to save them, but the question is: are they going to want to listen to him?

'Wendi's Magical Voice' is published by The Stuttering Foundation and written by Brit Kohls. Many children feel a bit nervous on the first day of school. Wendi the witch is no exception

She avoids speaking in the Magic School and when asked to introduce herself she is fearful, angry and frustrated. While the other kids are practicing their tricks for the Magic Fair, she crawls under the sofa, hoping to be invisible. But one day she becomes friends with Peter the Troll. He urges her to use her magic skills, even though she stutters. This booklet is about the differences between children that make them unique. A set of worksheets based on the book about Wendy was also developed, entitled *'Companion for Wendy's magical voice*. These funny worksheets contain language and speaking activities and provide opportunities to discuss attitudes and feelings about stuttering.

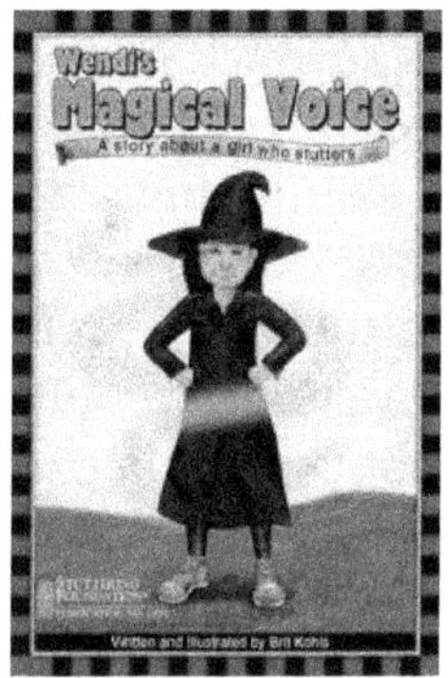

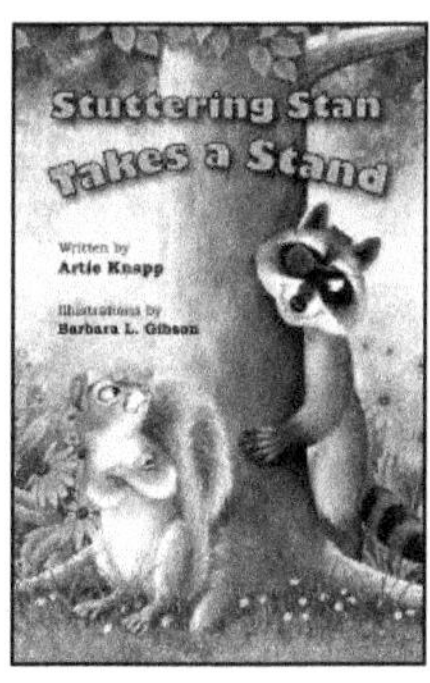

In the book *'Stuttering Stan Takes a Stand'* we follow Stan the squirrel, who is bullied because of his stuttering. He's afraid of arguing with his teasers up to the moment he makes a new friend who helps him understand that he's not the only one who's insecure. When Stan finally stands up for himself, he chooses to be kind and learns that friendship, understanding, and self-esteem are very important to everyone. This is how he brings all his friends together. A book that is not only about stuttering, but is also about dealing with bullying and teasing. For children between 5 and 10 years old.

'When Oliver Speaks!'" is written by Kimberly Garvin & Saadiq Wicks. It is an inspiring story about a boy with many talents and interests, who also happens to stutter.

That is why he does not want to give a speech in front of the class and always postpones it. With the help of his mom, he gets to work to deal with his stuttering and take on the challenge. It is worth mentioning that Saadiq Wicks is 13 years old and the founder of 'L-L-let Me Finish', a non-profit organization dedicated to support young people who stutter and to raise awareness about stuttering.

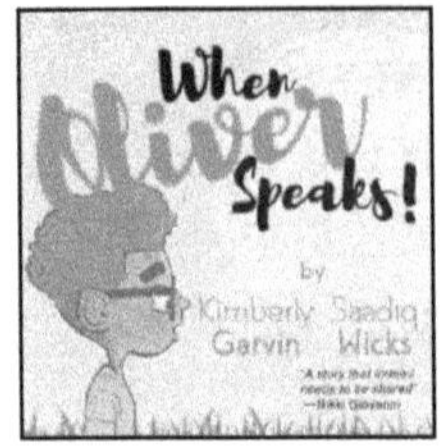

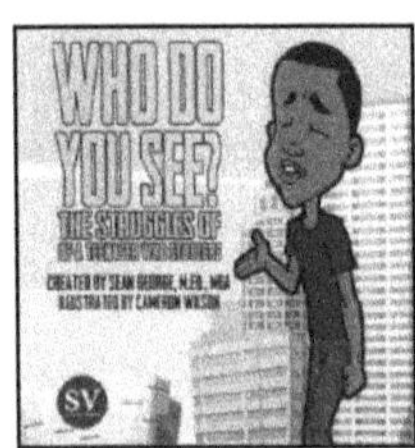

'Who Do You See? The Struggles of A Teenager Who Stutters' was written by Sean George, with illustrations by Cameron Wilson. The purpose of the book is to describe the different types of prejudices, stereotypes and misconceptions that teens experience daily because of their stuttering. The story also deals with a mother, who encourages her son to focus less on what others think of him and more on his own future.

Eric Kahn Gale wrote *'The Zoo at the Edge of the World'*. Marlin is a friendly, empathetic guy of 13 years old, who, because of his severe stuttering, has a very difficult time communicating with other people. However, he finds it very easy to talk to the animals of the jungle zoo that his father, who is an explorer, founded in the wilderness of Guyana in the late 19th century. Marlin finds that he has the gift of not only talking to the animals, but also understanding them. He discovered this special gift after he met a beautiful jaguar, the latest acquisition of the zoo. It's a story that resembles the theme from *'A boy and a jaguar'* described above. For children from 7 to 8 years old.

Vince Vawter's *'Paperboy'* is a multi-award winning children's book. The story is set in 1959. The narrator, Paperboy, takes over his friend's newspaper round while on vacation. Dropping the papers isn't a problem - he is known as one of the best pitchers in baseball - but he's bored and concerned about how,

The protagonist tells the story in short paragraphs, which summarize the way he imagines speaking fluently, without commas, because there are enough pauses in his speaking. Over the weeks, his stuttering improves slightly and eventually he even manages to pronounce his own name, which starts

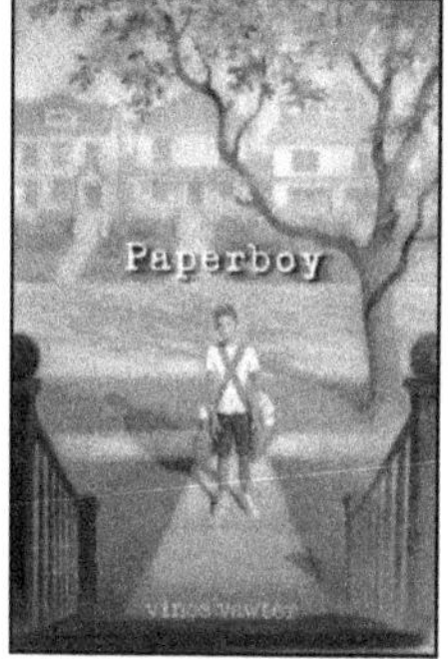

with the letter, which is the most difficult of all for him. Jane Fraser, President of the Stuttering Foundation of America, said about this book: “Paperboy offers a penetrating look at both the mystery of stuttering and the everyday frustrations that accompany it. Readers of all ages will appreciate the positive and universal story”. For young people from 10 to 12 years old.

C-C-C-C-Cornelia Thornhill, from Kimberly Newton Fusco's book *'Tending to Grace'*, stutters

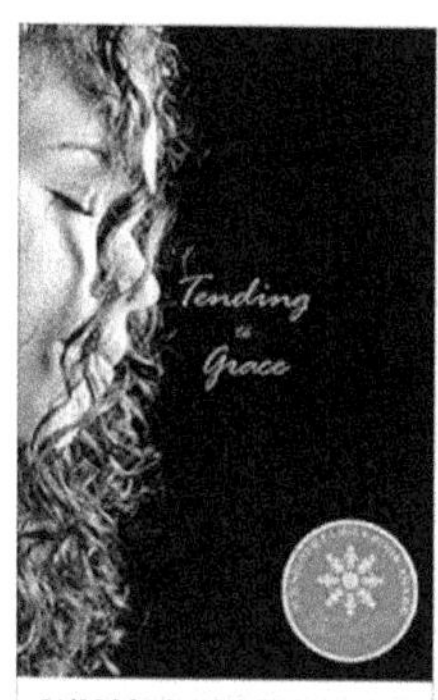

uncontrollably. She is a neglected child who does not talk to anyone. She keeps things going at home, since her mother Lenore is completely incalculable and irresponsible. Then her mother suddenly leaves for Las Vegas together with her boyfriend and she drops her daughter at Aunt Agatha's, who is actually a stranger to her. Cornelia bottles up her feelings and still refuses to speak. Then she finds out that she is actually smarter than she thought. She meets a girl, Bo, who has a father who is a bogeyman and who refuses to let his daughter go to summer class to learn to read.

Cornelia takes it upon herself to teach her that. However, when Bo's father finds out, he gets very angry, but Cornelia defends herself and her friend. In this way she breaks through her silence and learns to stand up for herself. For children and young people from 12 to 15 years old.

Films and music

In films we find a lot of characters who have problems speaking fluently. As far as English-language films are concerned, we find a nice overview in the article by Bruti and Zanotti (2018). These authors state that, in addition to sensory impairments such as deafness and blindness, stuttering is also fairly frequently represented in films and on television. While stuttering is sometimes used to represent ways of personal growth, the condition is much more commonly used to portray a character as psychologically weak or morally reprehensible. Moreover, PWS are often presented as unreliable. In other cases they endanger the lives of others through their clumsiness, in still other cases their stutter is a shield to hide their deceitful or malicious nature. A third function, associated with stuttering, is to provoke laughter, even tending towards the farcical, as we will also see in the operas mentioned below. In general, this leads, in most cases, to the creation of maladaptive and regrettable stereotypes designed to influence public perception.

Evans and Williams (2015) investigated whether the negative and stereotypical image that exists in public opinion about stuttering and PWS could indeed be found in films and whether, in line with other limitations, a turn towards a more positive portrayal had occurred in more recent years. Their results were disappointing. Of the 40 films that featured PWS they watched and rated, only three were found to paint a positive picture of people who stutter. They were often portrayed in a comic role, experiencing little joy in life (both in connection with their work situation and on a relational and family level) or as "broken" in one way or another (social, mental or moral). Evans and Williams conclude that their research confirms the largely negative characterization of PWS and that unfortunately no real shift in a positive direction was noticeable.

An important exception to the usually negative connotations regarding stuttering and PWS is the film *'The King's Speech'*. Kuster (2011) wrote an article about this film with the striking title "At long last, a positive portrayal of stuttering". According to her, this film has had a major influence on public opinion with regard to (people who) stutter, if only because of the overwhelming media attention.

'The King's Speech' is a 2010 historical drama directed by Tom Hooper, based on true facts. Colin Firth plays the role of the future King George VI in a very masterly way. The king makes an appeal to Lionel Logue, an Australian speech-language therapist (role by Geoffrey Rush). The two men become friends as they work together. When his brother renounces the throne, the new king leans on Logue to get him ready to give his first radio speech in 1939, in which England declares war on Germany. By the way, Logue was in the studio during the speech to support his royal patient. Screenwriter Seidler inquired about the life of George VI after he himself overcame his stuttering problem, which he had suffered from childhood. He began writing about the relationship between the therapist Logue and his royal patient in the 1980s, but at the request of the Queen Mum, he pledged not to publish it until she died, which happened in 2002. Afterwards he rewrote the scenario for the theater, focusing mainly on the relationship between the two men. Nine weeks before filming began, Logue's notebooks were discovered, allowing some of his quotes to be included in the script. It goes without saying that PWS and therapists view this film with a critical eye (Kuster, 2011). After all, some of the views on stuttering, and especially on its treatment, seem strange today. It should therefore be realized that the film is set in the 1930s and 1940s. Things like "putting

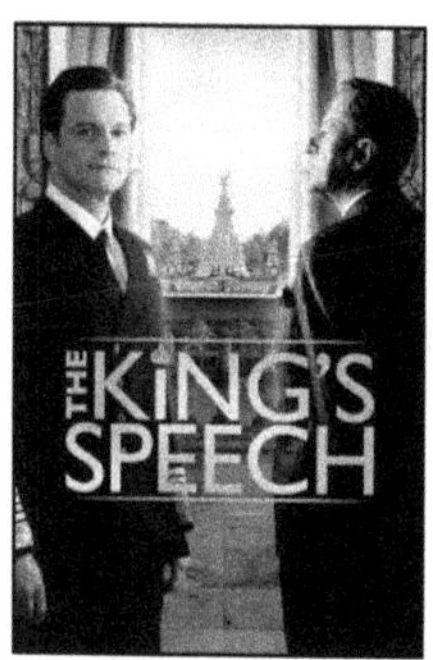

marbles in your mouth", "smoking to relax the throat" are, of course, unthinkable nowadays. The idea that stuttering is caused by forcing a left-handed person to become right-handed or that stuttering is due to strict upbringing has also been abandoned today. On the other hand, Logue pays a lot of attention to motivation and a good therapeutic relationship, which is still essential now. A number of "fluency-shaping" techniques (masking, singing, talking loudly, ...) are also discussed in the film. Although the king did not get rid of his stuttering completely, he learned to communicate quite efficiently.
Regarding the rather negative representations of PWS, Bruti and Zanotti make a distinction between on the one hand films, in which PWS are presented as a comic element, and on the other, those that portray them more as dramatic characters. In the latter category, they make a further distinction between stuttering as a sign of weakness, recurring stuttering and feigned or simulated stuttering. We give a few examples of each of these categories.

One of the oldest films in which a stuttering character is portrayed as comical is the 1935 cartoon *'Porky Pig'*. The reason for this is that the voice actor, Joe Dougherty, himself had a serious stuttering problem. Because he had difficulty controlling his speech, the recording sessions sometimes took hours and production costs were high. Dougherty was eventually replaced, but Porky continued to stutter, including using compensation strategies. At a certain point he wants to ask what is happening. "What ha-ha-..?" becomes "What's going on?". One of the 1937 cartoons featuring Porky is even entitled *'The Case of the Stuttering Pig'*. Johnson (1987) made an analysis of Porky Pig's stuttering behavior and found that the pig stuttered on as much as 23% of its words.

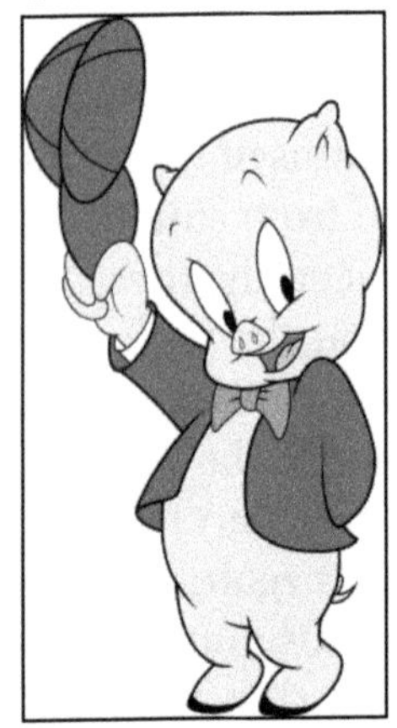

Perhaps the best-known film featuring a PWS is *'A Fish Called Wanda'* from 1988 (director Charles Crichton). The character Ken Pile is played by Michael Palin, a member of the Monty Pythons. John Cleese, who wrote the scenario, also plays one of the leading roles. Although Ken is the right-hand man of the criminal George Thomason, he is a very timid and reserved person who loves animals. After playing this role, Palin agreed to give his name to "The Michael Palin Center for Stammering Children" in London, a specialized center that does research on stuttering and provides treatment for children who stutter. Palin's involvement is certainly also related to the fact that his father suffered from stuttering. This personal experience gave him a model for playing Ken. Although the film is entertaining and funny, it does contain scenes in which he is severely harassed for his stuttering or in which the dysfluencies are so pronounced that they become almost dramatic[8]. There are also times when Ken does not stutter, e.g. when he is comfortable or furious. At the end of the film, he retaliates against Otto (played by Kevin Kline), who tortured him and ate some of his favorite fish. Suddenly he realizes that he no longer stutters and he tests himself by trying a tongue twister: "Hey! I've lost my stutter. It's gone. I can speak. How much wood could a woodchuck chuck,. . . if a woodchuck could chuck wood".

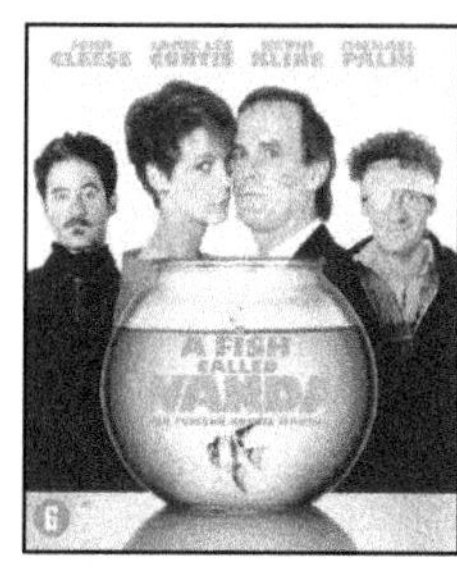

The movie *'My Cousin Vinny'* is a 1992 American film comedy directed by Jonathan Lynn. In the film, two young New Yorkers, who are passing through rural Alabama, are arrested for a murder they did not commit. First, they are defended by their cousin Vincent "Vinny" Gambini, who doesn't make much of it. They lose their confidence in his competence and

[8] For an example: https://www.youtube.com/watch?v=fSu5W0BtXG8

therefore engage a certain John Gibbons. This one is a very talented lawyer, but the good performance of his job is greatly compromised by a serious stuttering problem, which is very striking in his opening statement. The man's speech problem is presented in a very extreme way, including head movements and other secondary behaviors[9].

Woody Allen made the movie *'Broadway Danny Rose'* (1984), in which he also plays the lead role. Danny is an impresario and one of his clients is Barney Dunn, a stuttering ventriloquist. This one is portrayed as an absurd, weird man, a loser, even booed by 4-year-old children.

There are many other examples of films in which stuttering, often in a rather vulgar way, is only used to achieve comic effects (Johnson, 2008). For example, Mel Tillis, who himself stuttered for life and was best known as a country singer (see later), uses his speech problem to induce laughter in films such as *'Cannonball Run'*, *'The Villain'* and *'Smokey and the Bandit II'*, in which he always plays a supporting role. It is important to underline that if the stutterer is used purely as a comic figure, he or she is not a representation of a person, but is actually only presented as the embodiment of his speech problem. The only intention is that he/she stutters and therefore serves to amuse.

Now let's look at some PWS, who are portrayed as dramatic characters in movies. Often these are portrayed as weak personalities. Billy Bibbit (role of Brad Dourif) in Milos Forman's 1975 movie *'One Flew Over the Cuckoo's Nest'*, based on Kesey's book (see earlier) offers a prototypical example of a dramatic, stuttering character. Billy is a shy, anxious, psychiatric patient.

---

[9] See for a fragment: https://www.youtube.com/watch?v=mSw9_bsTzkU

A similar dramatic depiction of a PWS is found in Philip Kaufman's 1983 semi-autobiographical film *'The Right Stuff'*, which tells the story of the pilots selected for the Mercury Project, the first US manned space flight program. One of those pilots is John Glenn, the first American astronaut to orbit the Earth. The film focuses on his wife, Annie, who is portrayed as a very timid person with a serious stuttering problem. She is introduced in a scene, alone with her husband, in which she literally fights to get her words out. Another pivotal scene is where we see the car of the vice president, Lyndon B. Johnson, parked at the Glenns' house and Johnson, with the cameras in his wake, asking to be let in to meet her. When she refuses, a NASA official urges John Glenn to call her and convince her to let the vice president in. While still on the phone, she fights with her words and her emotions, revealing the external characteristics of her stuttering behavior (grimaces, movements,...). Annie Glenn, who died in 2020 at the age of 100, was awarded the First National Award by the American Speech and Hearing Association (ASHA) in 1983 for her unwavering commitment to individuals with communication disorders. In 1987, the "National Association for Hearing and Speech Action" presented the first annual "Annie Glenn Award" to a person who, despite having a communication disorder, distinguished him/herself exceptionally in society.

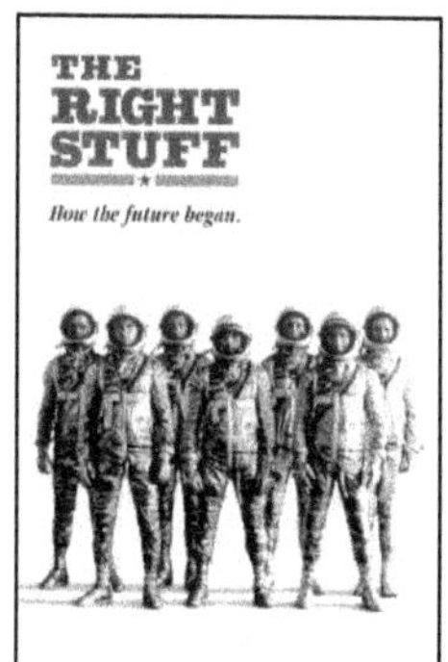

In the film *'Do the right thing'* (1989, directed by Spike Lee), one of the supporting roles is played by Smiley, a young, mentally weak man with a serious stuttering problem, who tries to make a living through selling photographs of Malcolm X and Marin Luther King.

The 1999 film *'The Hurricane'* (directed by Norman Jewison) is about Rubin "Hurricane" Carter. The lead role is played by Denzel Washington. It is the true story of the world-famous boxer, who was innocently arrested and convicted of triple murder in 1966. There was massive protest and many ordinary people, but also artists, athletes and musicians campaigned for his release (see among others the protest song 'Hurricane 'by Bob Dylan). He was only released in 1988, after the appeal court ruled that he had not received a fair trial. Carter himself said in an interview about his stuttering problem: "I have actually been in prison all my life. I was a violent stutterer from childhood and that was my prison. It was my stumbling, bumbling tongue that would not allow me to function in a group. When people laughed with me, the only sound they heard was my fist zooming through the air." This physical response from Carter is somewhat comparable to the one we described earlier regarding the sailor Billy Budd in Melville's story. Anyone who cannot be proven right verbally sometimes does so in a physical, violent way. For a further description of this phenomenon we refer to Harison (2011).

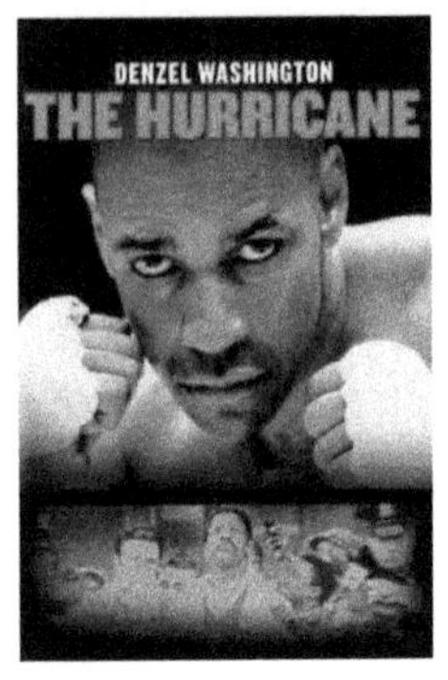

Marie is a little girl with a stuttering problem in the movie *'Paulie'* (1998, directed by John Roberts). When she starts getting speech therapy for her problem, her parrot begins to talk too.

In the beautiful film *'Dead Poets Society'* (Peter Weir, 1989), Tod is a shy, stuttering boy who is urged by Mr. Keating (role of Robin Williams) to push his boundaries and to speak at the front of the classroom.

An archetypal depiction of a stuttering boy can be found in the character Bob in the film *'The Cowboys'* (Mark Rydell 1972). The film tells the story of Will Anderson (role played by the legendary John Wayne), an elderly rancher who hires some schoolboys to help him bring his cattle to the market. One of the boys, Bob, has a serious stuttering problem, which prevents him from warning Will that one of the other boys is in great danger of drowning when he falls off his horse while crossing a river. Will is furious and the following conversation unfolds:

> WILL: You there! You almost killed him, you know that?
> BOB: But I t-t-t-tried to tell you.
> WILL: Yes, you did!
> BOB: I r-r-r-really tried.
> WILL: If you would have been lying there in that water, we would have heard you.
> BOB: I c-c-c-couldn't get the w-w-w words out.

A similar situation occurs in the movie *'Pearl Harbor'*, in which Red Winkle, who stutters severely, tries to warn his fellow soldiers that the Japanese attack on Pearl Harbor is starting and fails to do so because of his stuttering. We see close-ups of Red gritting his teeth and blinking as he tries to speak.

In the 1998 film *'Urban Legend'* (directed by Jamie Blanks), a scene occurs where a stuttering gas station attendant is unable, due to his speech impediment, to warn a customer that there is a murderer with an ax sitting in the back of his car.

We mentioned earlier that Stephen King's book *'It'* was being made into a TV series by Lawrence Cohen and Tommy Lee Wallace (1990). The stuttering of main character "Stuttering Bill" plays a prominent role. His fluency problem is a central element in his typing and is therefore often reflected in the dialogues.

A number of films feature people who have overcome their speech problem, but whose stuttering behavior flares up again (Bruti & Zanotti, 2018). Examples include: *'Dead Again'* (Kenneth Branagh 1991), *'The Sixth Sense'* (M. Night Shyamalan

1999), and *'J. Edgar'* (Clint Eastwood 2011). The observable symptoms of stuttering surface at crucial moments because of emotional tension or stress ('J. Edgar', 'Dead Again') or as a result of supernatural forces ('The Sixth Sense').

In *'The Sixth Sense'*, the one who stutters is a teacher, Stanley Cunningham, who was bullied as a child by his peers because of his speech problem, but who has overcome his stuttering. In one of the key scenes, Cole Sear, a deranged boy who can talk to the dead, addresses the teacher as "Stuttering Stanley," the name he was teased with as a child. While the whole class is shocked and silent, Cole goes on and says, "You spoke weird when you went to school. You spoke weird until you went to university". Controlled by a supernatural force, Cole calls out the nickname several times more, leading to Master Cunningham losing all control of his speech, so that his stuttering returns.

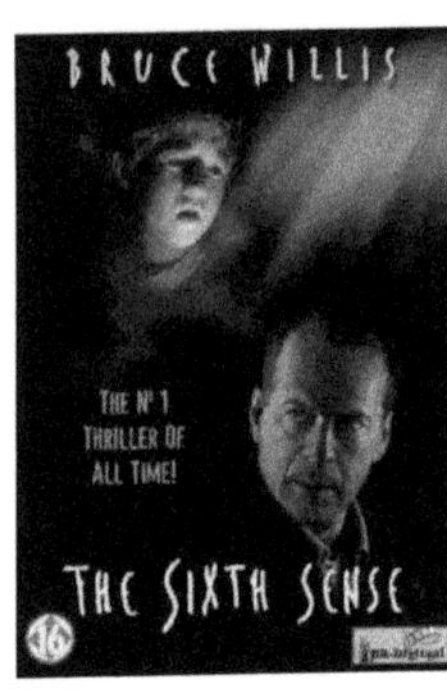

The idea that stuttering is a problem that can be overcome is central to the film *'J. Edgar'* by Clint Eastwood (2011). FBI chief J. Edgar Hoover learned to master his speech problem by teaching himself to speak very quickly, which even earned him the nickname "Speed." This suppressed stuttering, which led to a special way of speaking, characterized by exaggerated intonation and carefully controlled diction, is masterfully reconstructed in the film by Leonardo di Caprio. However, at times of great tension or stress, the stuttering behavior reappears. In a very dramatic scene with his dominant mother, where he confesses to her that he doesn't like women, he starts to stutter badly again.

A third subtype within the category of dramatic stuttering is feigned or simulated stuttering, which can be compared in a certain sense with simulated deafness (see further). Sometimes there is an explicit focus on the fact that the stutter was just a pretext, while in other cases it is left to the audience to deduce things for themselves. Usually, however, it coincides with the film's denouement.

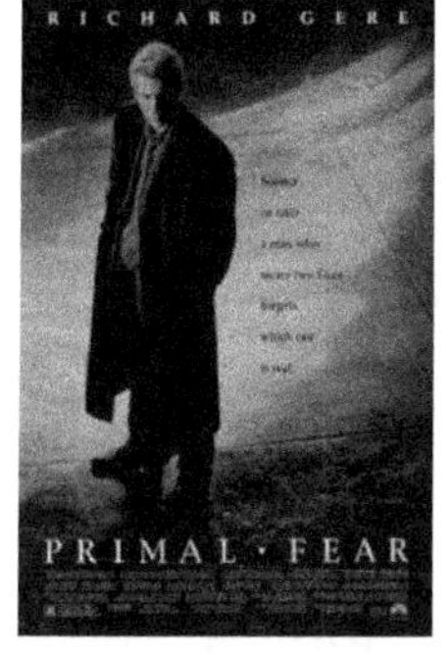

In the 1996 thriller *'Primal Fear'* (directed by Gregory Hoblit), Aaron (strong role by Edward Norton) is a homeless street child who is very shy and stutters. First he is protected by Archbishop Rushman, but then he is accused of the gruesome murder of the bishop. In prison he is examined by a psychologist, but he turns into his alter ego Roy and attacks her. This Roy is an aggressive, dirty-mouthed sociopath, who shows no trace of dysfluency. His attorney (role of Richard Gere) cannot act on Aaron's plea until he finds a way to reveal his client's dual personality. When cross-examined during the process, timid Aaron changes again into the aggressive Roy and physically assaults the prosecutor. He is therefore locked up in a high-security psychiatric ward. At the end of the film, however, he confesses that everything was faked and puts an end to his hypocrisy. The astute, confident Aaron admits that he did not simulate Roy's personality, but rather Aaron's. Only by pretending to be a stuttering weakling could he win the sympathy of his lawyer and the jury.

In the movie *'Harry Potter and the Philosopher's Stone'* (Chris Columbus 2001), it is one of secondary characters who pretends to stutter. Professor Quirinus Quirrell is a half-blood wizard. On his first meeting with Harry, Quirrel says, "Harry P-p-potter. I can't tell you how happy I am to meet you". In the end, Professor Quirrell's true nature emerges and he mentions his simulated kindness and his feigned stuttering.

Simon is a character from the movie *'Die hard with a vengeance'* (John McTiernan, 1995). He pretends to stutter to make the police believe he is a weak opponent. After all, they assume that someone who stutters, while trying to intimidate them, cannot possibly be a "hard one."

Finally, we mention two French film productions related to stuttering. *'Le bègue aimant'* (the Loving Stutterer) is a French short film (25 min.) from 2015, realized by Fabrice Roulliat. In the film, the young, charming Matthias dreams of winning the heart of his colleague Chloë. To do this, however, he must learn to deal with his greatest complex, namely his stuttering.

'La Façon de le dire' (The Way to Say it) is a French TV movie, made by Sébastien Grall in 1998. Nicolas is a PWS who is unable to overcome his speech problem. Folded back to himself, he maintains a correspondence with a young unknown woman. When she calls, he asks his brother to speak to her. But when she reports that she wants to come over and visit him, he panics. At that moment his grandmother tells him about an alternative therapy method, about which she saw a report on television and through which he would be released from his stuttering in a few days. Nicolas urges his mother to be allowed to follow this therapy. Just in time, through this revolutionary method, he succeeds in dissuading his brother from stealing his correspondence girlfriend. This film has been widely criticized for referring to the unprofessional, dubious and alternative method of treating stuttering it propagates.

Also in some operas characters who stutter play a role. One of the first of these was *'Il Giasone'* by Francesco Cavalli, an opera that was very popular in the 17th century. The plot is based on the story of Jason and the Golden Fleece, but a lot of comic elements have been added. The stuttering dwarf Demo also fitted in that context (Oster, 2006). *'La Nozze di Figaro'* by W.A. Mozart also features a stuttering character, namely the judge Don Curzio. In his memoirs, Michael Kelly (aka Ochelli), who was the first to sing this role, writes that he convinced Mozart to let his character stutter, also with the aim of making the audience laugh.

More recently, in Jacques Offenbach's 1851 opera *'Les Contes d'Hoffmann'* (The Tales of Hoffman), we find a stuttering house servant in the person of Cochenille. In Bedrich Smetana's comic opera *'The Bartered Bride'* from 1866, the beautiful Marenka's parents are looking for a rich young man for their daughter. A marriage broker is engaged. The boy Vasek, the son of a wealthy landowner, is found as a suitor, but he appears to stutter. However, the girl has set her sights on the poor Jenik. The marriage broker offers Jenik money to sell the girl.

The previously discussed book *'Billy Budd'* by Melville was not only made into a film, but was also adapted for the opera by Benjamin Britten in 1951. In contrast to the previously described humorous roles assigned to PWS, Billy is a dramatic character in this opera.

Stuttering even appears occasionally in popular songs. This might seem a bit strange, as it is known that persons who stutter are often fluent when they sing. It is generally known that some well-known singers show a lot of stuttering moments when they have to speak, but not as soon as they are singing on stage. In the US the well-known country singer Mel Tillis was a notorious stutterer, who even wrote the autobiography *'Stutterin 'boy'* about his speech problems. Other examples are Carly Simon, who began stuttering severely when she was eight years old, and Ed Sheeran, who tried a variety of speech therapies to help with his speech problem.

One of the best-known popular songs, featuring stuttering, dates from 1917 and was popular with soldiers and sailors. The song tells the story of a certain Jimmy, who falls in love with Kathy. We quote a piece of the text:

> *Jimmy was a soldier brave and bold,*
> *Katy was a maid with hair of gold,*

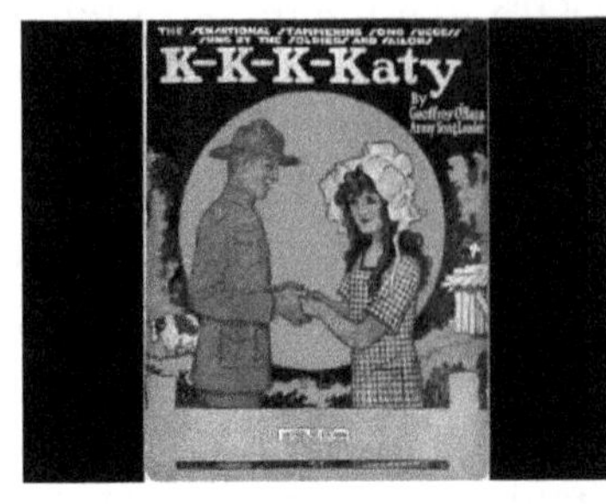

Like an act of fate, Kate was standing at the gate,
Watching all the boys on dress parade,
Jimmy with the girls was just a gawk,
Stuttered ev'ry time he tried to talk,
Still that night at eight,
He was there at Katy's gate,
Stuttering to her this love sick cry.

Refrain:
"K-K-K-Katy, beautiful Katy,
You're the only g-g-g-girl that I adore;
When the m-m-m-moon shines,
Over the cow shed,
I'll be waiting at the k-k-k-kitchen door."

Jimmy's stutter can't be explained by "shell shock" and thus by painful war experiences, as the man had yet to leave for battle. Perhaps it is a form of developmental stuttering, perhaps made worse by his shyness towards girls (Eagle, 2014). The full "sensational stammering song", composed by Geoffrey O'Hara, can be heard on you tube[10].

There are also a number of more recent songs, in which dysfluencies appear. A well-known example is "My Generation" by The Who, in which Roger Daltrey sings "Just talkin' bout my G-g-g-generation". Harison (2011) quotes Richard Barnes, friend and chronicler of the pop group, who may have been the first to state that this song with its stutter and its loud, violent final was particularly poignant and innovative. He wrote: "The Who turned "My Generation" into a biting, sarcastic tribute to

[10] see: https://www.youtube.com/watch?v=SAAkrI-aaOE

the youth, with phrases like "Hope I die before I get old". With his stuttered statements, a turned-up young person tells the older generation to get lost". Another example is the stuttering behavior in the 1974 hit song "You Ain't Seen Nothing Yet" by the group Bachman-Turner Overdrive. The stuttering ('B-b-b-baby, you just ain't seen n-n-nothin' yet ') was not supposed to be part of the final version, actually it was sort of a joke involving George, Randy Bachman's brother, who stuttered. Also in "Bennie & The Jets" by Elton John, also dating from 1974, stuttering appears.

Later, in 1995, stutterer Scatman John turned his problem into his strength and wrote the song "Scatman". By stuttering he created his own style of singing. His lyrics also proved to be inspiring for PWS, as the following lines show:

Everybody stutters one way or the other so check out my message to you
As a matter of fact, don't let nothin' hold you back
If the Scatman can do it, so can you.

References chapter 4

Block, K., Cameron, C. (2016). *Adventures of a Stuttering Superhero,#1. Interupt-itis.* Published by Kim Block.

Block, K., Cameron, C. (2018). *Adventures of a Stuttering Superhero,#2: Melissa Meets her Stamily.* Published by Kim Block.

Block, K., Cameron, C. (2019). *Adventures of a Stuttering Superhero,#3. Eye contact* Published by Kim Block.

Block, K., Cameron, C. (2020). *Adventures of a Stuttering Superhero,#4. Melissa stays home.* Published by Kim Block.

Brosch, S., Pirsig, W. (2001). Stuttering in history and culture. *Int. Journal of Pediatric Otorhinolaryngology*, 59;81-87.

Bruti, S., Zanotti, S. (2018). Representations of Stuttering in Subtitling. A View From a Corpus of English Language Films. In: Ranzato, I., Zanotti S. (Ed., 2018*). Linguistic and Cultural Representation in Audiovisual Translation*. New-York, Routledge.

Bushey, T., Martin, R. (1988). Stuttering in Children's Literature. *Language, Speech, and Hearing Services in Schools*, 19: 235-250.

Buwalda, P. (1999). *Het zal je kind maar wezen. Over Amerikaanse pastorale van Philip Roth.* De Gids,162;566-570.

Cabrera, A. (2001). Stuttering in literary arts. Retrieved on 20/01/2020 from https://www.mnsu.edu/comdis/isad4/papers/cabrera.html

Carroll L. (2018). *Alice in Wonderland.* Wordsworth Editions Ltd, Ware.

Cary, J. (2016). *The horse's mouth*. Thistle Publishing, London.

Conture, E. (2001). *Stuttering. It's nature, diagnosis and treatment*. Allyn & Bacon. Boston.

Cooper, J. (2007). *Autobiography of a stutterer*. BlazeVox books. Kenmore.

de Geus, E. (2011). *Sometimes I just stutter*. Stuttering Foundation of America, Memphis, Tennessee.

Down the rabbit hole and through the looking glass. The curious life of Lewis Caroll. *The Stuttering Foundation Magazine*, Fall 2020.

Duncan, M.H. (1949). Clinical Use of Fiction and Biography Featuring Stuttering. *Journal of Speech and Hearing Disorders*, 14, 139-142.

Evans, J., Williams, R. (2015). Stuttering in film media – investigation of a stereotype. *Procedia Social and Behavioral Sciences*, 193; 337.

George, S. (2019). *Who Do You See? The Struggles of A Teenager Who Stutters.* Independently published

Gerlach, H., Subramanian, A. (2016). Qualitative analysis of bibliotherapy as a tool for adults who stutter and graduate students. *Journal of Fluency Disorders*, 47, 1-12.

Harison, C. (2011) Redemptive violence and stuttering across the Atlantic: The Who's "My Generation" and Herman Melville's Billy Budd in historical perspective, *Atlantic Studies*, 8 (1); 49-68.

Hughes, J. (2014). *Steggie's stutter*. Windmill Books, London.

Jezer, M. (2008). *Stuttering: A Life Bound Up in Words*. Small Pond Press, London.

Johnson, G.F. (1987) A Clinical Study of Porky Pig Cartoons. *Journal of Fluency Disorders*, 12; 235 – 38.

Johnson, J.K. (2008). The Visualization of the Twisted Tongue: Portrayals of Stuttering in Film, Television,and Comic. *The Journal of Popular Culture*, 41 (2); 245-261.

Kahn Gale, E. (2015). *The Zoo at the Edge of the World*. Balzer & Bray/Harperteen, New York.

Kesey, K. (1962). *One flew over the Cuckoo's nest*. Viking, New York.

King, S. (1986). *It*. Viking, New York.

Knapp, A, Gibson, B. (2010). *Stuttering Stan Takes a Stand*. MightyBook Inc., Boston.

Kuster, J.A. (2008). Stuttering in Contemporary Literature. Last update 2008, retrieved from https://www.mnsu.edu/comdis/kuster/Bookstore/literature.html

Kuster, J.M. (2011). At Long Last, A Positive Portrayal of Stuttering. *ASHA Leader*,16 (2) Iss. 2, (Feb 15, 2011): 13,24-25.

Kohls, B. (2010). *Wendy's magical voice*. The Stuttering Foundation, Memphis, Tennessee.

Lears, L., Ritz, K. (2000). *Ben has something to say*. Albert Whitman & Co., Atlanta.

Lewinsky, C. (2019). *Der Stotterer*. Diogenes, Zurich.

Lewis, N. (2013). *Jackdaw Cake. An Autobiography*. Eland Publishing Ltd., London.

Logan K.J., Saunders Mullins, M. Jones, K.M. (2008) The depiction of stuttering in contemporary juvenile fiction: implications for clinical practice. *Psychology in the Schools*, Vol. 45(7); 609-626.

Melendez, J. (2018). *Easy For You To Say Stuttering*. Rare Bird books, Los Angeles.

Melville, H. (1924). *Billy Budd, Sailor: An Inside Narrative.*:Constable & Co, London.

Mishima, Y. (2000). *The Temple of the Golden Pavillion.* Everyman's Library, London.

Mitchell, D. (2006). *Black Swan Green.* Random House, New York..

Mitchell, D. (2011). Lost for words. *Prospect Magazine*, nr 180.

Muller, P. (2012). "The impediment that cannot say its name". Stammering and trauma in selected American and British texts. *Anglia*, 130; 54-74.

Myers, J. (2005). *Somerset Maugham: A Life.* Random House, New York.

Nina, G. (2019). *Stutterer Interrupted: The Comedian Who Almost Didn't Happen*. She Writes Press, Phoenix.

Oster, A. (2006). Melsima as Malady: Cavalli's Il Giasone (1649) and Opera's earliest stuttering roles. In: Lerner, N., Straus, J. *Sounding off: theorizing disability in music.* Routledge, p. 157-172.

Preston, K. (2013). *Out with It: How Stuttering Helped Me Find My Voice.* Atria Books.

Pudney, J. (1976). *Lewis Carroll and His World.* Scribner, New York.

Scott, J., Smith, S. (2020). *I Talk Like a River.* Neal Porter Books, New York.

Shields, D. (1989). *Dead languages*. Knopf publishers, London.

Somerset Maugham, W. (1991). *Of human bondage*. Bantam Classics, New York.

Spurr, D. (2011). Stuttering Joyce. *European Joyce Studies, 20,* 121-133. Retrieved February 14, 2021, from http://www.jstor.org/stable/44871324

Tillis, M. (1984). *Stutterin' Boy : The Autobiography of Mel Tillis.* Rawson Associates, London.

Trotter, W., Silverman, F. (1976). The stutterer as a character in contemporary literature: a bibliography. *Journal of Speech and Hearing Disorders*, 41 (4); 553-54.

Updike, J. (2012). *Self-Consciousness: Memoirs.* Random House, New York.

Van Riper, C. (1972[5]). Speech Correction. Principles & Methods. Constable, London.

Vawter, V. (2013). *Paperboy*. Random House, New York.

Warren, R.P. (1996). *All the Kings' Men*. Harcourt Brace, San Diego (first published 1946).

Waugh, E. (1945). *Brideshead Revisited.* Chapman and Hall, London.

Chapter 5: Mutism

Mutism can be described as the absence of any form of speech, whether spontaneous, in response to questions or imitative (Lafosse, 1998). Mutism often has a psychological cause, but it can also be the result of brain damage. There are different forms of mutism. Selective mutism sometimes occurs in children, while in adults we find post-traumatic mutism from time to time.

Selective mutism (SM) can be described as a mental disorder in children. Although the spoken language abilities are intact, we find a constant refusal to speak in certain situations or to certain persons (Witters & Manders, 1999). The first symptoms usually appear in infancy and the problem is more common in girls than in boys. Selective mutism is generally classified as a social anxiety disorder. Sometimes a distinction is made between selective and elective mutism. In the latter, the person concerned speaks in virtually no social situation, while in selective mutism it's about specific situations, such as not talking in class. However, the terms are often used synonymously.

Reactive mutism is a form of mutism that occurs as a result of one or more traumatic events (for example, a rape or a death). Children (or adults) who show this form are often moderately to severely depressed, lack social contacts and often show little or no facial expression (Van Borsel, 2010). As we will notice, it is striking how often this type of mutism occurs in stories.

Post-traumatic mutism, belonging to the category of post-traumatic stress disorders, is often associated with "shell shock" and can actually also be considered a form of reactive mutism. The term "shellshock" was first used in association with the First World War. Already during the first winter of that war, there were indications of a large number of mental breakdowns in hospitalized soldiers and officers. By 1916, 40%

of those injured in the combat zones were suffering from shell shock, and by the end of the war some 80,000 cases had passed through the British Army medical services. Paralysis, blindness, deafness, mutism and limping were most prevalent among the common soldiers, whilst nightmares, insomnia, palpitations, dizziness, depression and disorientation were more common among the officers. Although it was first thought that shellshock, as its name suggests, was directly related to close-up firefights and bombardments, it later turned out that soldiers further away from the frontline could also be involved. Mutism and other speech disorders, including stuttering, were among the most common forms of war neurosis. One possible line of thinking is that they were symptoms of suppressed aggression of the soldiers towards their superiors. After all, soldiers were supposed to remain silent and carry out the orders of their superiors, although in practice these sometimes amounted to suicide squads. Rather than cursing, slapping, or shooting their supervisor, they bit their tongues, distorted their speech, or kept completely silent (Leed, 1979).

We find examples of most of the above described forms of mutism in books and films. Nevertheless, we find references to selective and reactive mutism much more often than to the more specific post-traumatic forms, such as caused by the above mentioned war conditions.

(Auto)biographies and non-fiction

The reference book '*Can I tell you about Selective Mutism?*' was written by Maggie Johnson and Alison Wintgens. It is intended for family, friends and professionals. It contains a lot of accessible information and is an ideal introduction to selective mutism.

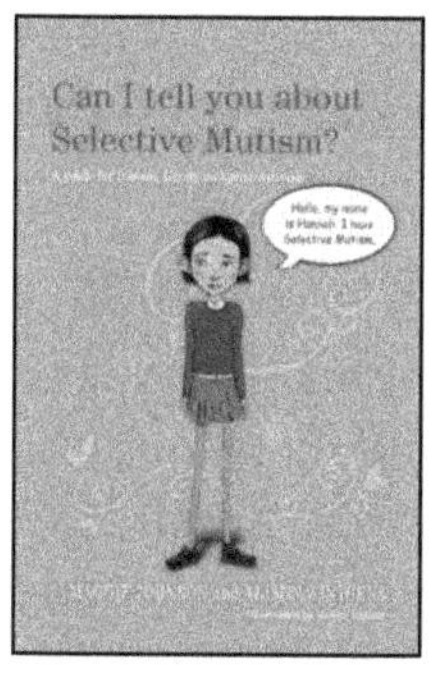

The book is dedicated to Hannah, a young girl with selective mutism. It invites the reader to learn about selective mutism from his/her perspective, help him/her understand what it is, what it feels like to have selective mutism and how best to help.

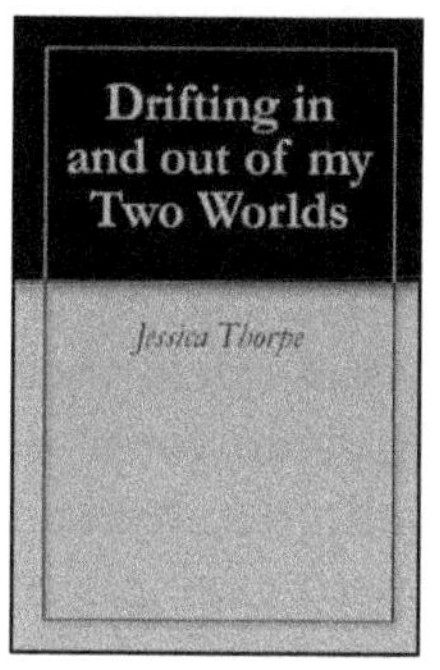

Jessica Thorpe's *'Drifting in and out of my Two Worlds'* is the fascinating story of a girl with Selective Mutism. It is based on true facts and on the real experiences of someone who has gone through it all herself and overcame her problem. It examines the great contrast she experiences between life inside and outside school, the total ignorance about the disorder, how to best deal with the problem and the profound consequences it can bring about if it is left untreated.

'Selective mutism in our own words' was written by Carlton Sutton and Cheryl Forrester. It's a book that can be seen as an eye-opener with very enlightening stories of people living with selective mutism. In this book, a number of people with selective mutism talk about their own experiences, in their own words, as the title indicates.

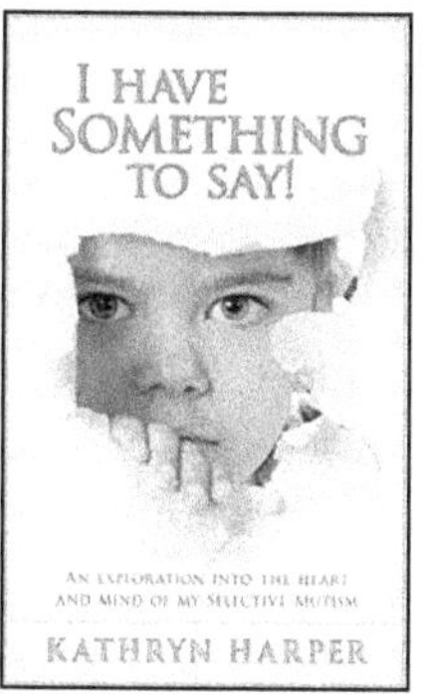

'I Have Something to Say!' by Kathryn Harper is subtitled 'An exploration into the heart and mind of my selective mutism'. The author suffered from selective mutism herself as a child, at a time when very little was known about this often misunderstood condition. In her teens and as a young adult, she developed a number of complications from the untreated anxiety disorder. In this book she wants to look back at her own past and let readers share her perspectives and

experiences, in order to create more and better insight and to generate more understanding for people who suffer from this disorder.

'Schuyler's Monster: A Father's Journey with His Wordless Daughter' is the story of a girl named Schuyler, written by her father Robert Rummel-Hudson. When Schuyler is 18 months old and not yet talking, her pediatrician tries to find an explanation for this. She is diagnosed with bilateral perisylvic polymicrogyria, an extremely rare neurological disorder caused by a brain malformation. Once her parents knew she couldn't (learn to) speak, they started looking for a way to help her learn. It is the story of a father and a mother who learn to deal with the limitations of their child. Today Schuyler can communicate with alternative and supported means of communication. In contrast to most of the works described above, where we are dealing with a psychogenic form of mutism, this is therefore a form of organically determined mutism. Actually we could also catalog this as an example of 'childhood anarthria' (see chapter 3).

Fiction

In *'The House of the Spirits'*, arguably Chilean Isabel Allende's best-known book, one of the main characters, Clara Trueba, sinks into mutism for years after witnessing her sister's sexual assault and the following autopsy. She keeps watch over the dead body all the time. Allende describes it like this (p. 47):

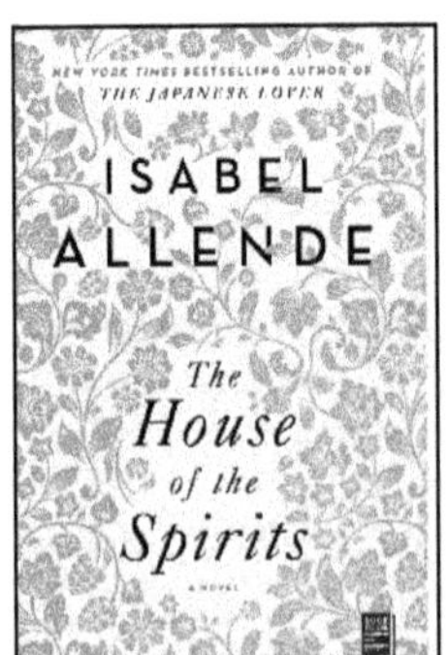

"She couldn't get away from that place until it got light. Then she crept back to her room. Silence took hold of her. She was absorbed in a world of silence and did not speak again until nine years later she raised her voice to announce her wedding ".

We can consider this as an example of the above described reactive mutism.

Julia Cunningham wrote a trilogy about a boy suffering from mutism titled *'Burnish me bright', 'The silent voice' and 'Far In The Day'*. The story is about Auguste, who does not talk and who is maltreated and abused as a servant. He escapes and takes refuge with Hilaire, a retired mime artist. Auguste is amazed at what Hilaire can do and he learns from him how to communicate without words.

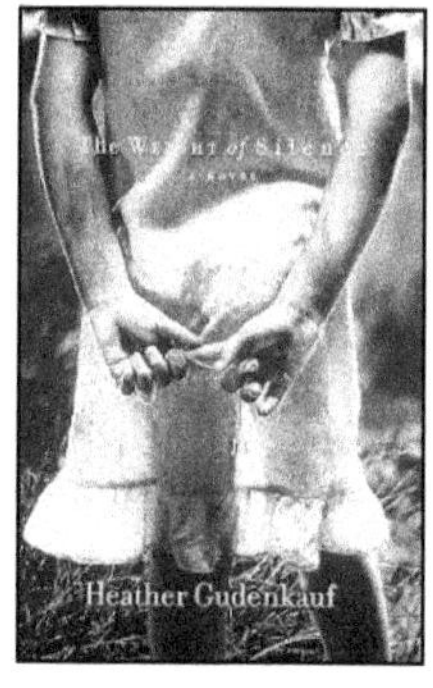

The multi-award-winning book *'The Weight of Silence'* was written by Heather Gudenkauf. One morning in August, two families wake up to find that their daughters have disappeared during the night. Seven-year-old Calli is a sweet, dreamy girl who suffers from selective mutism as a result of a tragedy she experienced as a toddler. Calli's mother, Antonia, has always sought to be the best mother possible within the confines of her marriage to a generally absent and often aggressive husband. Although she thinks her husband has nothing to do with the disappearances, she now fears that her decision to stay with her husband will cost her more than just her daughter's voice.

In Lois Lowry's 2005's *'The Silent Boy'*, the girl Katy is intrigued by a boy named Jacob, a calm, quiet guy who has a special relationship with animals, with whom he communicates through sounds and movements. Although Jacob never speaks to her, they nevertheless develop an unusual friendship and a mutual understanding for each other. The villagers find Jacob strange and a bit retarded, but Katy thinks he is at most a bit special.

''Halo: Ghosts of Onyx' is a science fiction novel written by Eric Nylund based on the Halo video games. The book features a female officer, Lucy-B091, who for years suffers from post-traumatic mutism after having witnessed her entire unit being destroyed.

One of the few books describing post-traumatic mutism due to "shell shock" is *'Regeneration'*, the first part of Pat Barker's magnificent WW-I trilogy. It deals in detail with the rehabilitation of physically, but especially also psychologically war-damaged British soldiers, who are being treated at the specialized "Craiglockhart War Hospital" in Edinburgh. One of the characters from *'Regeneration'* is Billy Prior. He is a soldier who suffers from mutism and asthma. According to some critics, Billy's inability to speak represents the way Western culture deals with the mutilation of soldiers' bodies during the war. Some of the soldiers at the military hospital, like Billy, are so traumatized by their horrific wartime experiences that they are unable to speak. Their muteness is a physical manifestation of the inability to process the horror of the things they experienced. Mutism therefore represents the repression of unspeakable, unbearable trauma and symbolizes the horrendous conditions and suffering of soldiers fighting World War I.

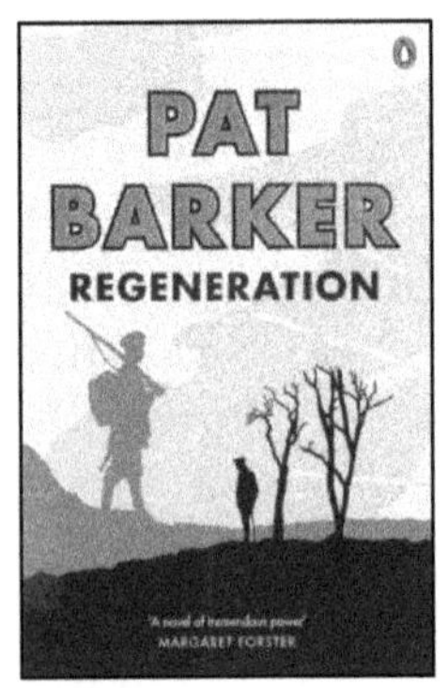

Prior is a working class officer who has worked his way up to being a lieutenant despite his humble background. Fighting himself with this class distinction, Billy notices that this is nevertheless also extended into the trenches. As a result, he constantly fights with himself: the struggle between his workers' origins and his army career, his longing for peace and at the same time the anger he feels towards the citizens, who have escaped the horrors of war and the trenches. We cite a small fragment (p. 55):

> Sister Rogers came back. 'Thank you. Now I just want to have a look at the back of your throat.
> 'Again the pad came out. 'THERE'S NOTHING PHYSICALY WRONG.'
> 'Two l's in "physically", Mr Prior. Open wide.
> 'Rivers drew the end of the teaspoon, not roughly, but firmly, across the back of Prior's throat. Prior choked, his eyes watered, and he tried to push Rivers's hand away.
> 'There's no area of analgesia,' Rivers said to Sister Rogers.
> Prior snatched up the pad. 'IF THAT MEANS IT HURT YES IT DID.'
> 'I don't think it hurt, did it?' Rivers said. 'It may have been uncomfortable.
> "HOW WOULD YOU KNOW?'
> Sister Rogers made a clicking noise with her tongue.

Like mutism, stuttering can also be a soldier's physiological manifestation of the inability to confront and talk about his terrible experiences fighting the war. It can be another representation of the human mind's inability to process the traumatic horrors of war. This was the case, among others, with the well-known war poet Wilfred Owen, who, like his fellow poet Siegfried Sassoon, was treated for a while in Craiglockhart. The character of the stuttering Septimus Warren Smith, described by Virginia Woolf in her book '*Mrs Dalloway*' (1925) is assumed by many to be based on poet Siegfried Sassoon. Septimus Smith shows a post-war neurosis and presents with hallucinations, tremors and stuttering.

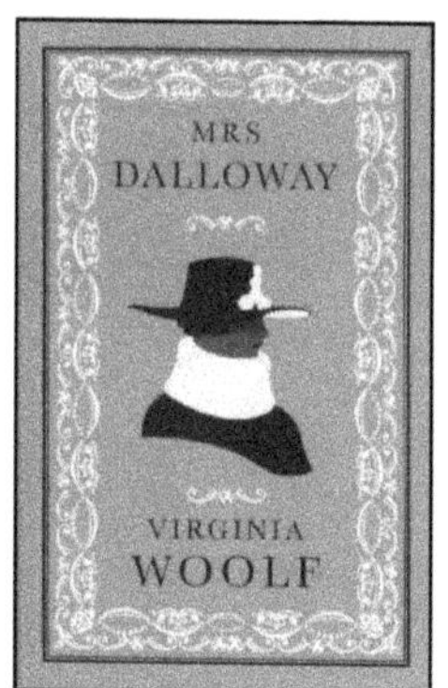

Children's books – young adult

We found some books, meant for children, parents and educators, dealing with (selective) mutism.

In Wen Wen Cheng's *'Maya's voice'*, Maya is a bright, curious girl who likes to let her beautiful voice be heard. But when she first goes to school, she loses the confidence to use her voice and doesn't say anything all day. With a lot of time, patience, understanding and love of her surroundings, she eventually rediscovers her voice. For 4 to 8 year olds.

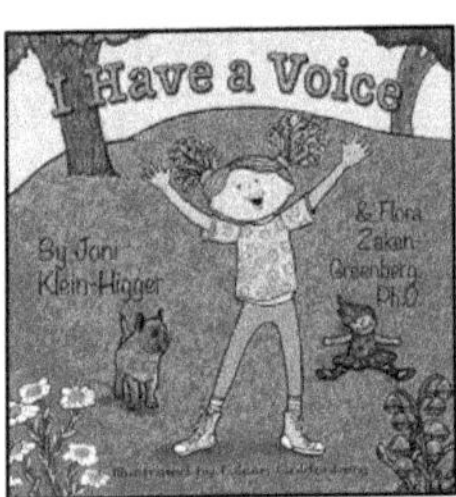

'I have a voice' was written by Joni Klein-Higger. The story is about Jamie, who is attending kindergarten for the first time. However, she has a big problem... she does not dare to speak. Mama takes her to Dr. Faye, who not only teaches her to talk, but also stimulates her self-confidence to overcome her fear. For children 3 to 6 years old.

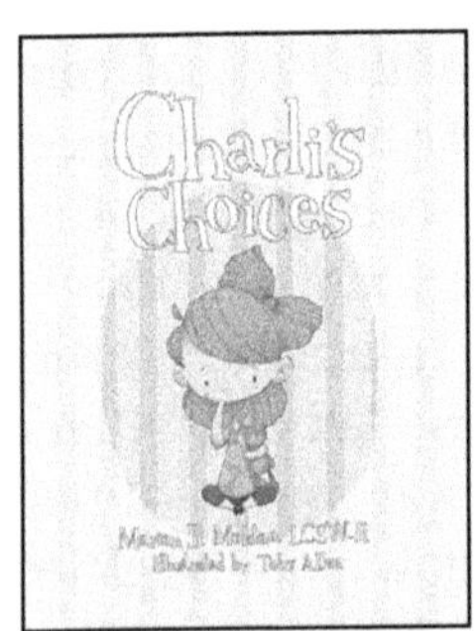

In *'Charli's Choices'* by Marian B. Moldan, Charli never says a word except at home. She only speaks to her father and her mother and even when grandma and grandpa come over, it takes a long time before she says anything. This booklet is inspired by the author's many years of experience working with children who have selective mutism and/or are socially anxious. It supports children with this problem as well as their parents and educators.

Sam, the giraffe, loves trucks, dogs and chocolate, but all people know about him in school is that he rarely, if ever, talks.

He has prepared a very good presentation, but is afraid to deliver it in front of the class. Eventually he does it anyway and the other kids learn a lot more about him. The next time he has to speak in class, things will be much better. The booklet *'Too shy for show-and-tell'* was written by Beth Bracken and is intended for children aged 4 to 6 years.

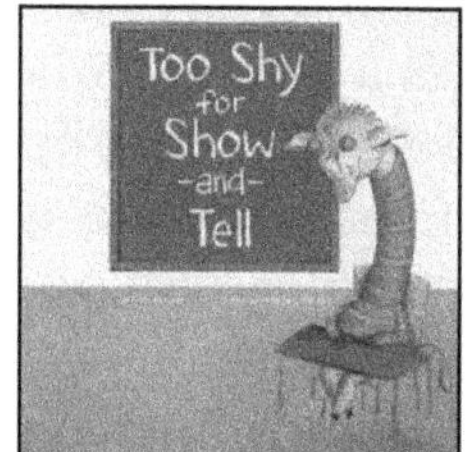

In Tom Neely's booklet *'Mary-Ellen O'Keefe's Word-Speaking Diet'*, Mary-Ellen O'Keefe is a wise and happy little girl who loves to talk, sing, ask everyone out and blurt out anything that comes into her head. Things change on her first day of school. The new, unfamiliar environment makes her nervous and shy and puts her on an unexpected and peculiar "word diet." It was as if her mouth had been glued. The teacher and the other children cannot find out what kind of child Mary-Ellen really is. With the help of her mom and her teacher, she eventually gets out.

Sharon Longo's *'My friend Daniel doesn't talk'* is about the friends Ryan and Daniel. The extrovert Ryan befriends Daniel, who is afraid to talk at school and anywhere else except at home. Ryan defends his friend through thick and thin. Eventually, Daniel feels confident enough to speak to Ryan. Ryan's tendency to talk too much helps Daniel in the classroom, but still he hopes that one day Daniel will be able to speak in the classroom in front of the others, so that they can find out who he really is. For children from 9 to 12 years old.

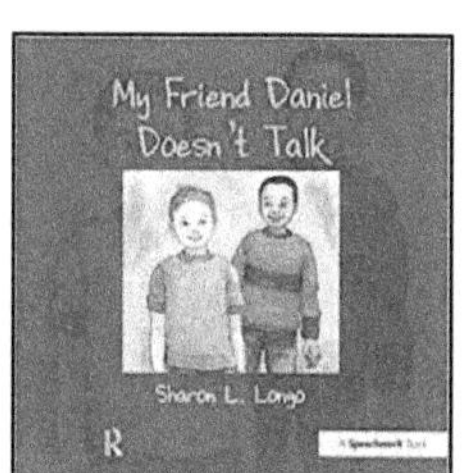

'Silence is Goldfish' by Annabel Pitcher is about Tess, who discovers that her father, Jack, is not her real, biological father. At that moment she becomes silent. With a silent protagonist, there are few dialogues in this story. Tess only talks to a goldfish-shaped flashlight. In the end, "all's well what ends

well", when Tess forgets the search for her real father at the moment she realizes and experiences how much Jack loves her.

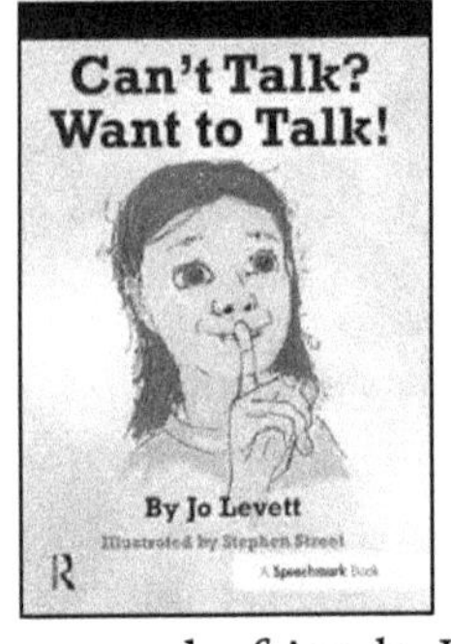

Jo Levett wrote the book *'Can't Talk, Want to Talk!'*. When Lily meets a little girl who is too scared to talk at school or other places outside her house, she is friendly to the quiet girl. Their friendship grows, and the quiet girl feels comfortable enough to talk to her new friend. This is an illustrated storybook for children with Selective Mutism to learn them that, like Lily, they can make friends. It is also a useful resource for parents, friends and teachers of children with SM to understand why these children are unable to speak in some circumstances and how to develop certain strategies to reduce their fear of speaking.

The following books are written for young adults.

John Marsden's book is titled 'So *much to tell you'*. The target age category is from about 13 years on. The story, partially based on true facts, goes like this. Well before the start of this book, Marina has been the victim of a marital argument that got out of hand. She suffers from her injuries, does not want to speak anymore and shuts herself off from the outside world. After admission to a psychiatric hospital, she is placed in a boarding school, where she gradually feels at home and is accepted. Starting from that situation she feels strong enough to contact her father (who has mutilated her). With the help of diary fragments, the writer brings the girl to life with her problems and daily worries. Her emotional life, problems and doubts are expressed in a convincing way. Only when she comes face to face with her father, she speaks her

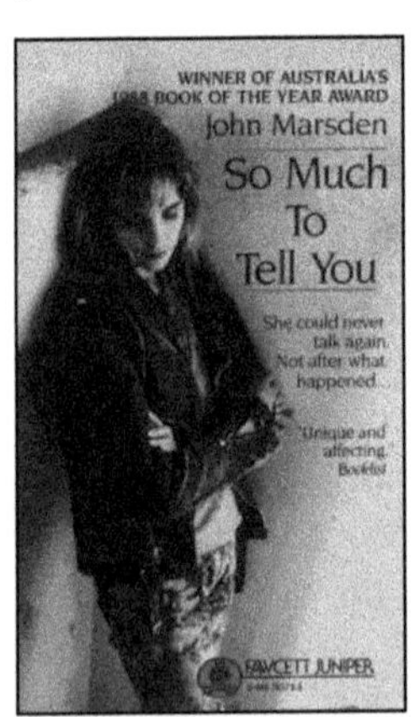

first and in the book also the last words, from which the novel takes its title: "Hello, Dad... I've got so much to tell you...".

Sara Barnard's *'A Quiet Kind of Thunder'* is about Steffi and Rhys. As long as she knows, Steffi has selective mutism. This makes her feel invisible. But Rhys, the new kid at school, sees her. He is deaf and, because Steffi knows some sign language, she is assigned to take care of him. It doesn't matter to Rhys that she doesn't speak, they will find other ways to communicate. Ultimately, Steffi finds her voice again. For youngsters from 13 to 14 years on.

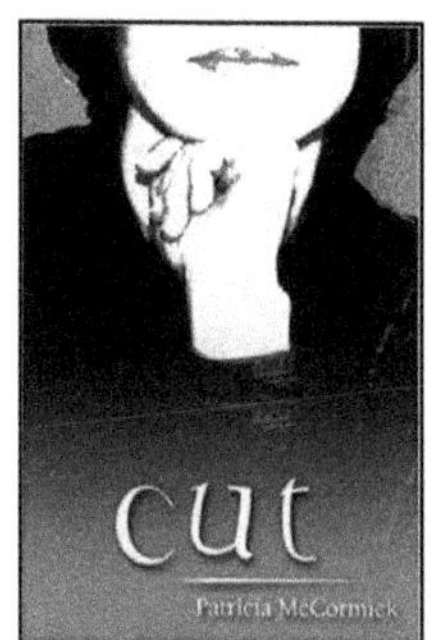

In Patricia McCormick's book *'Cut'*, the main character, 15-year old Callie doesn't speak to anyone, not even to her therapist at the treatment center where she has been admitted, after her parents and the family doctor have discovered that she mutilates herself. Finally she does start talking to her therapist/doctor who helps her understand why she cuts herself. She regains her voice and eventually dares to face the trauma that has provoked her behavior. Intended for young adults (13-17 years old).

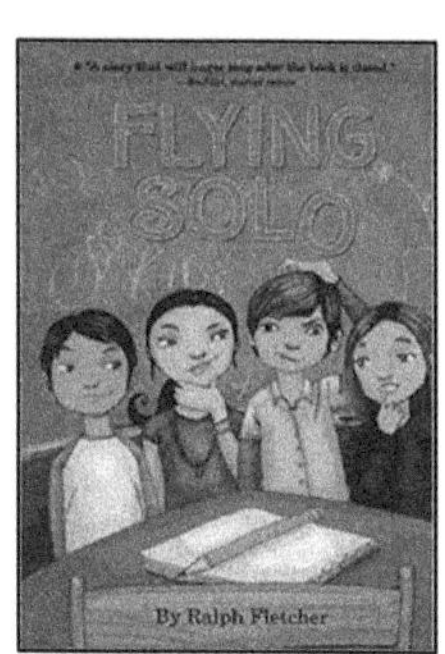

In the book *'Flying Solo'* by Ralph Fletcher (2008), an incredible opportunity arises one day in teacher Fabiano's sixth grade. The teacher is absent and no replacement shows up. The class wants to prove that "KIDS RULE" is a valid statement and thus they decide to run the class themselves. Super-smart Karen takes the lead and most of the kids participate. But for Rachel it's not just any day. It has been exactly six months since their classmate Tommy died and since then Rachel has stopped speaking and communicates only by writing notes. In her own way she points this out to her classmates and for the first time they express their true and sometimes hurtful thoughts and feelings. How should things proceed now? After all, the school day is far from over. How is this going to end? For children from 12 to 16 years old.

'Silent to the Bone' (2000) is an award winning novel by E. L. Konigsburg recommended for 10-14 year olds. The story is told by 13-year-old Connor Kane. His best friend Branwell has turned to mutism and has been taken to a youth facility after his sister has suffered brain injury and has fallen into a coma. The au pair Vivian claims that Branwell has dropped his sister. Connor suspects that there must be some explanation for Branwell's silence, and that Branwell certainly did not injure his sister intentionally. He visits him every day, but because Branwell doesn't talk, they have to make do with a kind of sign language and with blinking, like Bauby in *'The diving bell and the butterfly'* (see earlier). Together with his older half-sister, Connor sets out to solve the mystery of why Branwell stopped talking and what really happened to his sister. Together with Connor Kane - who also does not shy away from confronting himself - the reader gets closer to the truth step by step, the true facts behind the testimony of the devious Vivian and the silence of the sensitive Branwell. Driven by a sense of shame about his adolescent crush on the au pair, he has never said anything about her misguided behavior and her lack of care for the baby and thus doesn't dare to speak. Based on a true story, recommended for ages 12 to 14.

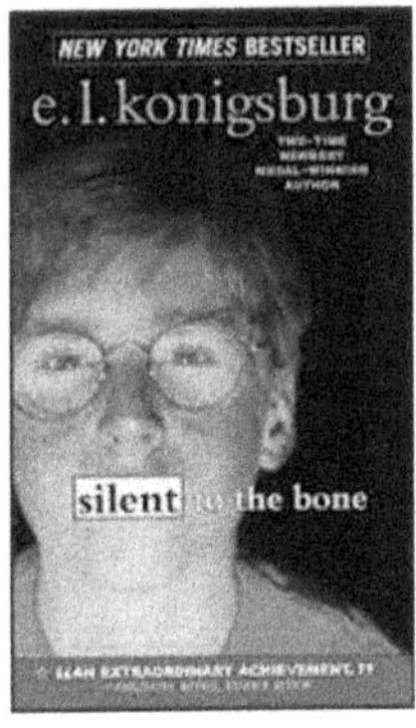

Films

A lot of short, but also somewhat longer documentary films about selective mutism can be found on the internet. As an example we mention the poignant British documentary *'Help*

Me To Speak - Selective Mutism'[11]. It follows two children with selective mutism, Rob and Madeleine, for a year.

'My Child Won't Speak'[12] (2009) is about three girls with the same problem.

'The Piano' is a 1993 **fiction film** directed and written by Jane Campion with a beautiful soundtrack by Michael Nyman. Ada (role of Holly Hunter) is a Scottish woman whose mutism is not caused by a medical condition, but

is due to a psychological incident when she was six years old. Since then she communicates only through her beloved piano and by using sign language, which is then translated by her daughter Flora. One day, Ada's father sends her with her daughter by ship to the other end of the world, to New Zealand, where she is married off to Stewart, a cool, distant settler. Once there with her daughter and her piano, Stewart decides to sell the piano to a certain Baines. This makes Ada so sad that she feels disgust for Stewart. Baines proposes that Ada can earn her piano back at a rate of one piano key per "lesson", provided that he can observe her and do "things he likes" while she plays. But there are also other conditions attached to this. At first she feels disgust for the man, but gradually she starts an intimate relationship with him. At the end of the film, she chooses to learn to speak again.

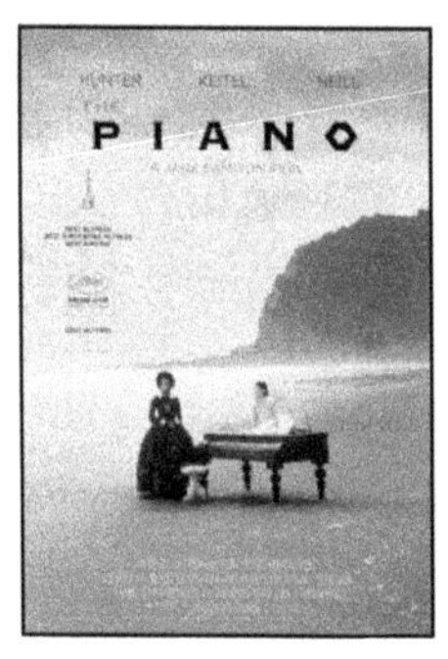

In the 1993 film *'House of Card'"* by director Michael Lessac, the 6-year-old girl Sally refuses to speak after her father passes away. The same phenomenon also occurs in the animation film *'The prophet'* from 2014, which is loosely based on the book by

---

[11] See the complete documentary at: https://www.youtube.com/watch?v=kkNtFpidYao

[12] Watch it on youtube: https://www.youtube.com/watch?v=toX0GLFbtiQ

Kahlil Gibran. The story takes place in Lebanon in Ottoman times. The widow Kamila works as a housekeeper for Mustafa, a poet, painter and political activist, who is under house arrest. He is guarded by the soldier Halim, who is secretly in love with Kamila. Kamila's daughter Almitra has stopped speaking after her father's death and has become a troublemaker, often stealing from nearby merchants. Her only friends are the seagulls, with whom she even seems to be able to communicate by making bird sounds herself.

The previously discussed book *'Regeneration'* by Pat Barker was both adapted for the theater by Nicolas Wright and for the silver screen by director Gillies MacKinnon (1997).

A recent film is *'Sibel'*, in which the main character is a young woman who has been unable to speak since she had a fever at the age of five. It is a 2018 German-Turkish film directed by Guillaume Giovanetti and Çagla Zencirci. When the inhabitants of the Turkish village, in which the film is set, have to communicate with each other over a greater distance, they do so in a kind of particular whistle language. Sibel masters this whistling as the best and uses it as a means of communication.

References chapter 5

Allende, I. (2011). *The House of the Spirits*. Vintage Books, New York.

Barker, P. (1991). *Regeneration*. Viking Press. New York.

Barnard, S. (2017). *A Quiet Kind of Thunder*. Macmillan Children's Books. London.

Bracken, B.(2014). *Too shy for show-and-tell*. Picture Window Books. Edina.

Cheng, W-W. (2013). *Maya's voice*. CreateSpace Independent Publishing Platform, Scotts Valley.

Cunningham, J. (1980). *Burnish me bright*. Dell Pub Co., New York.
Cunningham, J. (1983). *The silent voice*. Yearling, London.
Cunningham, J. (1980) *Far In The Day*. Dell Pub Co, New York.
Fletcher, R. (2008). *Flying Solo*. HMH Books for Young Readers, New York.
Gudenkauf, H. (2009). The Weight of Silence. Mira publishers, London.
Harper, K. (2015). *I Have Something to Say!: An exploration into the heart and mind of my selective mutism*. Green Cup Publishing, London.
Johnson, M., Wintgens A. (2012). *Can I tell you about Selective Mutism?* Jessica Kingsley Publishers, London.
Klein-Higger, J. (2016). *I have a voice*. Guardian Angel Publishing, Inc., New York.
Konigsburg, E.M. (2000). *Silent to the Bone*. Simon & Schuster, Bloomington.
Lafosse, C. (1998). *Zakboek Neuropsychologische Symptomatologie*. Acco, Leuven.
Leed, E. (1979). *No man's land. Combat and Identity in World War I*. Cambridge University Press, Cambridge.
Longo, S. (2006). *My friend Daniel doesn't talk*. Speechmark Publishing Ltd., London.
Lowry, L. (2005). *The silent boy*. Dell Laurel Leaf, London.
Marsden, J. (2004). *So much to tell you*. Walker books, London.
Moldan, M.B. (2014). *Charli'S choices*. Archway Publishing, Bloomington.
Newton Fusco, K. (2005). *Tending to Grace*. Laurel Leaf, New York.
Nylund, E. (2011).*Halo: Ghosts of Onyx*. Uitgeverij Tor, s.l. .
Pitcher, A. (2015). *Silence is Goldfish*. Hachette Childrens Group, London.
Rabinowitz, A. (2014). *A boy and a jaguar*. HMH Books for Young Readers, Boston.
Rummel-Hudson, R. (2008). *Schuyler's Monster: A Father's Journey with His Wordless Daughter*. St. Martin's Press, London.

Thorpe, J. (2013). *Drifting in and out of my Two Worlds*. Lulu publishers, London.

Van Borsel, J. (2010). Psychogene spraakstoornissen: een kennismaking. *SIGnaal*, 72; 22-39.

Witters, I., Manders, E. (1999). Selectief Mutisme: een literatuuroverzicht. *Tijdschrift voor Logopedie en Audiologie*, 29; 122-127.

Woolf, V. (1981). *Mrs Dalloway*. Harcourt, San Diego, New York, London.

Chapter 6: Hearing Loss and Deafness

Usually, one speaks of deafness when there is a hearing loss of more than 90 decibels. As soon as the hearing loss exceeds 30 dB, the term hearing loss is used. In the latter case, it is often possible to compensate for the hearing loss by means of a classic hearing aid, in case of deafness only an inner ear prosthesis (cochlear implant or CI) can help in a number of cases. Quite a lot of books have been written in which deaf and hard of hearing people appear. Moreover, they also very often figure in films. Nevertheless, Dakin (2009) states that in many books and films deaf and hard of hearing characters are only 'used' as a catalyst to initiate or accelerate a plot or to better emphasize the qualities and/or attitudes of the hearing persons. They are rarely used for who they are, for their own merits, not to mention a few exceptions.

We are aware that we had to make a selection for this chapter and that it will therefore be very incomplete, given the profusion of mentions in all kinds of media.

(Auto) biographical books and non-fiction

One of the most famous and a somewhat special autobiography on deafness is that of Helen Keller (1880-1968) entitled *'The story of my life'*. Keller became seriously ill as a toddler and then got both blind and deaf.

She had only a few memories of the visible world and of the sounds of everyday life. In her book she writes with humor and with some self-mockery about the unyielding nature that enabled her to develop her own script, learn to read, write and even study. It is a fascinating testimony from and about a woman who overcame her limitations to participate fully in life. Her life story was also filmed under the title *'The miracle worker'* (see below).

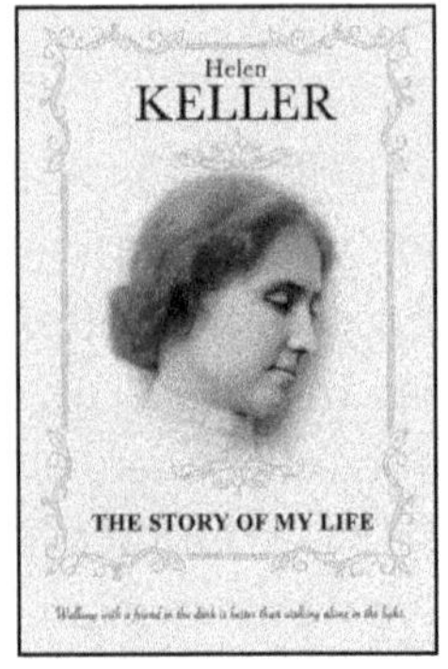

'Haben: The Deafblind Woman Who Conquered Harvard Law' by Haben Girma (2020) can be considered a present-day equivalent of Keller's life story, although there are of course some big differences.

Haben Girma was the first deafblind person to graduate from Harvard Law School. In this book she tells the story of her life so far in 24 short chapters, covering episodes from her childhood through her professional life. Being the daughter of Ethiopian/Eritrean immigrants, she grew up with very limited vision and hearing, growing even worse over the years. She developed new methods of communication. To give an example: she was the one who came up with the idea of carrying a wireless keyboard that would allow another person to type information that would be transmitted to her computer, equipped with a refreshable braille display. Haben became an advocate for the deaf and blind communities, working as a disability rights lawyer. In her book she also describes how she met with US President Barack Obama at the White House to highlight the importance of accessible technology. A story of courage and perseverance, but also told with a sense of humour.

'In silence. Growing up hearing in a deaf world' is the (auto)biographical story of a hearing daughter, whose parents are both deaf. Since her parents usually spoke in sign language, that also was Ruth's language until she was five. When she

went to school, she was therefore placed in a class for mentally retarded children. Enraged, Ruth's mother went to school to complain. Then a miracle came into the house, a radio, and

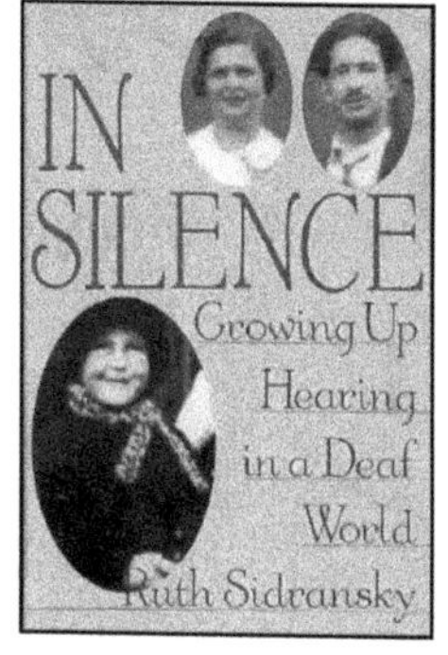

Ruth finally learned to speak. Yet she remained an outsider, unlike other children who had 'normal' parents. Ruth's memories of her childhood are joyful but also bittersweet. The loving bond with her parents was as fragile as the red ribbon that tied her to her mother at night as a baby, so Mother Mary could feel the movements of the child that she couldn't hear crying. She remained sort of trapped between two worlds: her own, quiet, safe world at home and the great, hearing, often cruel world outside. Thus young Ruth fought her struggle to find a place of her own.

In the Dutch language book *'Cochleaire Capriolen'* (Eng: Cochlear Capers) Elske Posthuma tells what it is like to be hard of hearing from birth on. Elske was struck by sudden deafness several times. With the last period of sudden deafness dating from October 2008, the hearing did not return. In April 2009 she underwent surgery and received a cochlear implant. After intensive rehabilitation, she could hear, listen and understand again. She tells what the consequences are if you miss a lot in your environment because you are seriously hard of hearing and what it is like to lose more and more of the wonderful experience of making and listening to music. This is the story of someone who, despite all the setbacks, continues to shape her ideals and make her dreams come true. With the help of the CI, Elske is now no longer deaf but hard of hearing again and is even hearing more than in the past thirty years.

Fiona Bollag, together with three co-authors, wrote in 2007 the book *'Das Mädchen, das aus der Stille kam'* (The girl who came out of the silence), being her own history as a girl who doesn't hear anything, or rather didn't hear nothing. She was born deaf and learned to read lips at a young age. At sixteen, however, she was one of the first to receive a cochlear implant, with which her brain can convert sounds, so that she can hear again. Suddenly, Fiona lives in a completely different world. Imagine how frightening it is to suddenly hear music or traffic rushing by overnight? Fiona describes in an intuitive way what a gift it is to be able to hear for the first time in your life, but also that the years in silence were a gift as well. Because with the CI it became clear that hearing involves a lot of things: background noises, emotions in voices, raindrops falling... Beautiful sounds, but also confusing and distracting sounds. Fiona's special story is worth to be heard: it is a positive note for anyone who has to live with a smaller or greater disability.

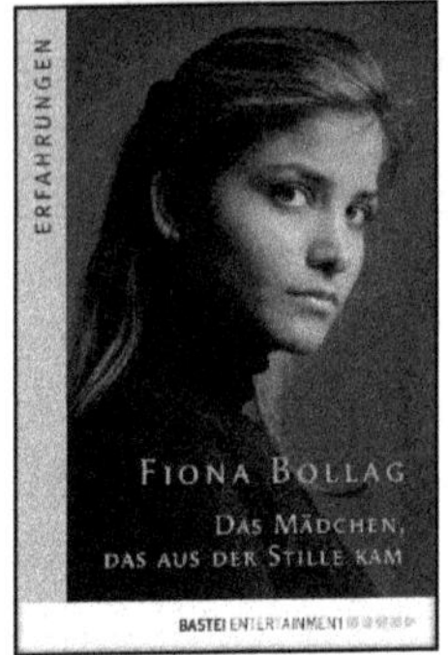

Stuart Blume is a sociologist. For years he has been following developments in medical science and technology with a critical eye. On May 24, 1989, this research suddenly gains an extra dimension. On that 'pleasant day of spring' what his wife Anja has suspected for some time is confirmed: their one and a half year old son Jascha is deaf. Confusion, sadness, guilt are the result. And the overriding question becomes: what should we do, what is best for this child? Blume, affiliated with the University of Amsterdam, is looking for the answers, as a scientist and as a father, and in the vague hope that the former can be of service to the latter. In the fascinating *'Grenzen aan genezen'* ('Limits to cure') he reports on that quest, in which he elaborates on CI and all the developments surrounding it.

The well-known neurologist Oliver Sacks wrote the book *'Seeing Voices. A journey into the world of the deaf'*. It's an essay about the deaf, their sign language and the social-emotional problems some of them experience. When Sacks came into contact with the deaf, a new world opened up for him: the brains of the deaf who grew up with sign language appear to undergo a completely different development than those of hearing people. They are often better developed in some respects, especially spatial. He was most affected by the life histories of deaf people and their struggle to break through the wall of silence and the misunderstandings that often surround them. The book consists of three parts, of which the second part is probably the strongest. Sacks constantly alternates the essay form with very personal semi-scientific treatises on the history of the education of the deaf, the importance of gestures and sign languages and also thoughts about language (philosophy) and thinking. Neurological processes are likewise given the necessary attention.

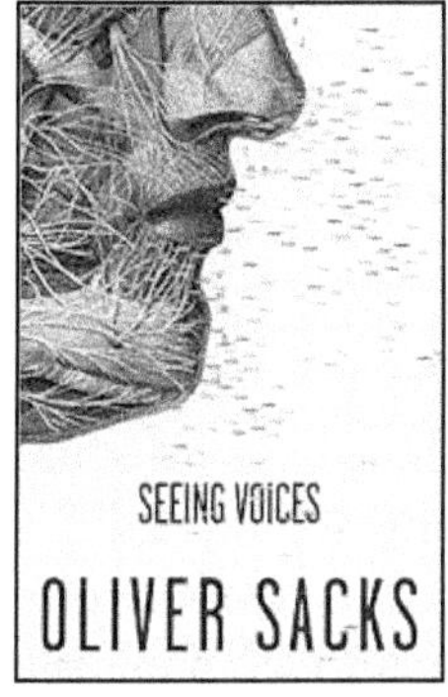

In the book *'A quiet world. Living with hearing loss',* David Myers, who himself experienced progressive hearing loss, explores the problems of hearing impairment both at home and at work, and provides information on new technologies and breakthrough surgical procedures. He further describes from his own experience how he has learned to deal with his hearing loss and how he brought in new technological tools to facilitate his life. Finally, he also gives tips and advice to family and friends regarding how to deal with people with hearing loss.

'Deaf Like Me' by Thomas and James Spradley is a moving account of parents trying to come to terms with the deafness of their baby daughter Lynn. The love, hope and fear of all hearing parents with deaf children are expressed in a simple, yet powerful way. In the epilogue, Lynn, now a teenager, reflects on her deafness, her upbringing, her struggle to learn to communicate, and the discovery that she was the subject of a book written by her father and her uncle.

Ruth Silver describes in *'Invisible: My Journey through Vision and Hearing Loss'* how she became not only progressively becomes more and more visually impaired due to retinitis pigmentosa, but how she also loses her hearing. Still Ruth refuses to surrender to the darkness and the silence. Inspired by her own experiences and challenges, she founded the "Center for Deaf-Blind Persons" in Milwaukee, USA, a non-profit organization dedicated to providing assistance to individuals with the dual disabilities of which she herself suffered. *'Invisible'* dispels myths, describes useful learning procedures, gives hope to people with these kind of disabilities and their families and also reassures fellow sufferers through her own example that people with severe disabilities can lead a rich and meaningful live.

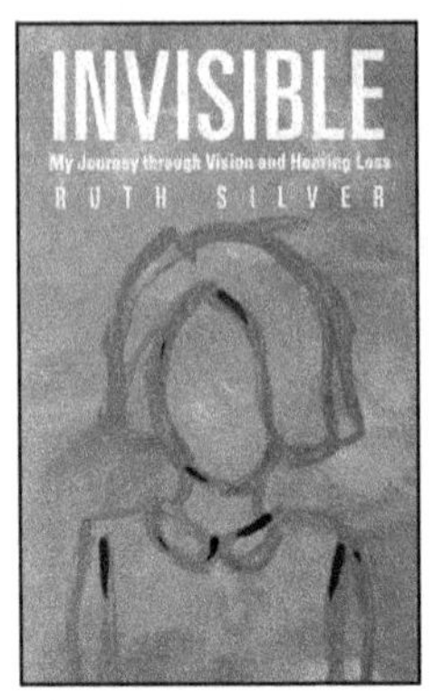

'The Cry of the Gull' (original French title : 'Le Cri de la mouette') is an interesting autobiography of the French actress Emmanuelle Laborit.

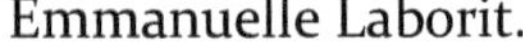

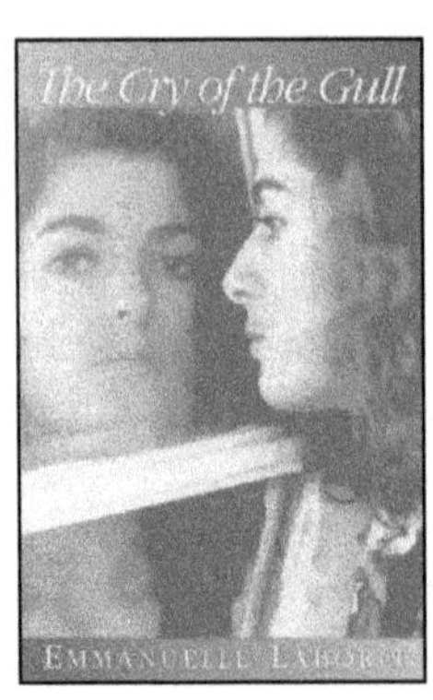

Emmanuelle was born in a small village in France. Her parents didn't understand why she did not learn to speak. When she was three years old, they decide to take her to a specialist, who immediately detects the little girl's deafness. Her mother then creates a real relationship of intimacy with her daughter while her father, especially because of his work but also because of his child's disability, has a more tense relationship with his daughter. One day, when Emmanuelle is seven years old, her father hears about 'sign language' on the radio. He takes his daughter to Vincennes to learn this language. She finally has a real identity. Later on Emmanuelle goes to Washington with her parents to discover the way of life of American deaf people. At the age of eleven, she enters sixth grade at the Morvan- school, that offers special education for the deaf and hearing impaired, but she discovers that it is forbidden to express herself in sign language. The young girl is outraged at having devoted so much effort to learning sign language and not being able to use it and, at thirteen, Emmanuelle decides to stop learning. Finally her parents discover that she is skipping school. She then promises them that she will never do it again and keeps her promise, but does nothing in class. She spends time on parties, cigarettes, alcohol and drugs, but after having crossed some boundaries, she stops doing stupid things. The young girl makes plans for the future, starts acting and plays a role in a film. She is offered a cochlear implant that will allow her to hear, but she refuses because she wants to stay as she is, and accept her difference. She then plays a role in the theater production *'Les Enfants du silence'* (the French version of *'Childen of a Lesser God'*, see below) and wins the 'Molière for theatrical revelation', becoming the first deaf person to win that prize.

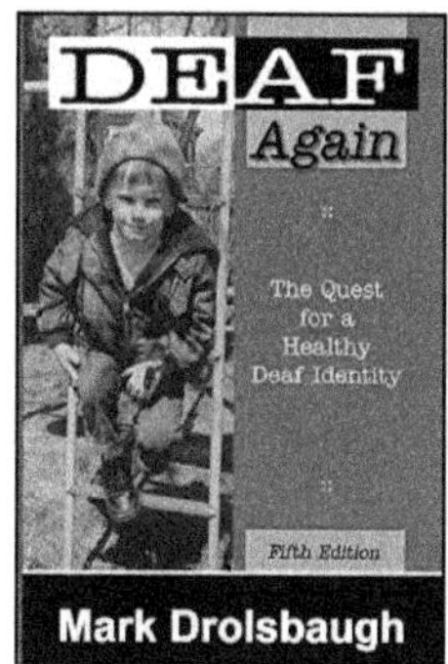

'Deaf Again' by Mark Drolsbaugh describes the fascinating journey of the author from hearing toddler... to hard of hearing child... to deaf adolescent... and ultimately, to culturally Deaf adult. The struggle to find one's place in the deaf community is challenging, as Drolsbaugh finds, yet there is one interesting twist: both his parents are also deaf. This book offers great insight and well-considered arguments on subjects like signing versus oralism and on cochlear implants. From the same author is the book *'Anything but silent'* (2004), that offers a good perspective of the world of deaf and hard of hearing people. We cite a quote from *'Deaf Again'* on the importance of communication:

> "Neither religion nor race mattered to me, but communication did. If you were willing to be my friend

and accept my deafness, I didn't care if you were white, black, Catholic, Jewish, Swahili, or whatever. I didn't care if you worked as a CEO or passed your time handing out flowers at the airport. If you can communicate, you're my friend".

'Hear Your Life: Inspiring Stories and Honest Advice for Overcoming Hearing Loss' contains a number of inspiring and enlightening stories of people with hearing loss and their way back to better hearing, brought together by expert Melissa Rodriguez. She also answers frequently asked questions about hearing loss and includes a guide full of useful information.

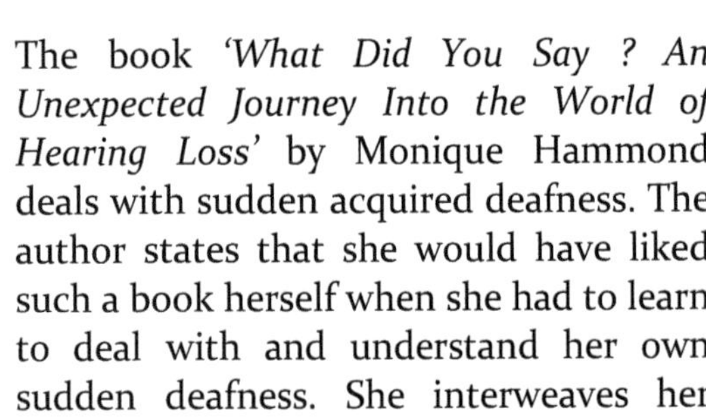

The book *'What Did You Say ? An Unexpected Journey Into the World of Hearing Loss'* by Monique Hammond deals with sudden acquired deafness. The author states that she would have liked such a book herself when she had to learn to deal with and understand her own sudden deafness. She interweaves her story with a wealth of information about causes and types of hearing loss, audiological research, hearing aids, self-help groups, etc. This book was written with a lot of wisdom and insight.

'Train Go Sorry: Inside a Deaf World' by Leah Hager Cohen depicts the story of students at a school for the deaf in New York City. The author, who is a hearing person, grew up on the school's campus, since her father was its superintendent. This book discusses various conflicting facts and attitudes that makes one's round regarding the education of the deaf, but without taking sides. The conflict between those who propagate American Sign Language (ASL) and others

preferring the oral method is well documented and the debate on cochlear implants is not avoided.

Fiction

Again we start again with classical, historical literature.

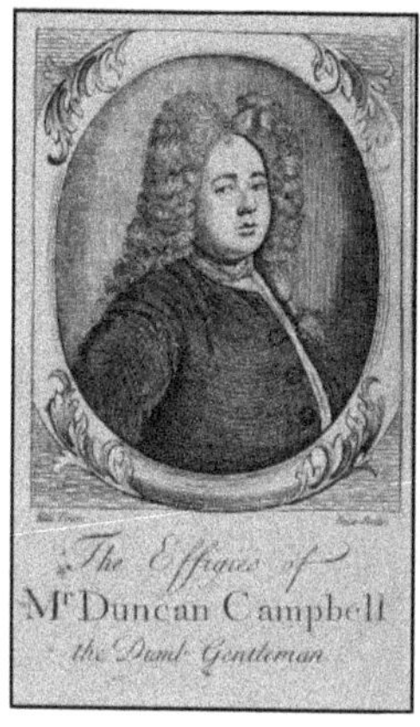

According to Dakin (2009), *'The life and adventures of Mr. Duncan Campbell'*, written by Daniel Defoe and published in 1720, is one of the first literary portraits of a deaf-mute person. The book tells the story of a man who, beneath his limitations, also had some very special gifts: at first sight he could write down the name of every stranger he encountered, he could predict the future, etc. Perhaps Defoe (best known for his book *'Robinson Crusoe'*) became interested in deafness through his brother-in-law, who had developed a method for the education of the deaf and who also laid the foundation of a system of fingerspelling, elements of which were later adopted in British Sign Language.

In an article in the leading magazine The Lancet from 1925 (!), Yearsley writes that in books and theater much more attention is paid to blindness than to deafness. He notes that when a blind person is performed in the theater, the audience is moved to tears, but that a deaf person appearing leads mostly to laughter. He argues that this is one of the reasons that so little attention is paid to deafness in fiction literature. We have to realize, however, that it only concerns books from before 1925. Yearsley mentions the book *'The Peveril of the Peak'* by Sir Walter Scott from 1823, in which a certain Fenella pretends to be deaf, *'The Virginians'*, by William Thackeray (1858) with the stone-deaf Lord Chesterfield, but especially two books by

Charles Dickens. In *'A tale of two cities'*, Miss Pross loses her hearing due to a pistol shot close to her ear.

However, it is in *'Dr Marigold'* (1865) that a deaf girl, Sophy, is described in detail. This Doctor (nick name) Marigold is a street vendor. One day he adopts a deaf-mute girl whose mother has died and who is constantly beaten by her real father. A nice excerpt is the description of Dr. Marigold's attempts to learn Sophy to read. We quote:

> "At first I was helped - you'd never guess by what - Milestones. I got some large alphabets in a box, all the letters separate on bits of bone, and saying we was going to WINDSOR, I gave her those letters in that order, and then at every milestone along the way, I showed her those same letters in that same order and then pointed to the abode of royalty. Another time I give her CART and then chalked the same upon our cart. Yet another time I gave her D-O-K-T-E-R M-A-R-I-G-O-L-D and hung a corresponding inscription outside my waistcoat."

Both become very attached to each other, but when she is 16 years old, Marigold thinks it is time to send Sophy to a school for the deaf-mute in London so she can learn more. This leads to an emotional goodbye, when the school principal asks him, "Will you be able to be separated from her for two years?" to which he replies, "Yes, if it works for her." The man then says, looking at Sophy: "There is also another question. Can she be without you for two years? ".

A few years before Dickens, Wilkie Collins had also painted a portrait of the deaf girl Mary in the book *"Hide and Seek.* Mary is nicknamed Madonna because of her beauty. She is also rescued from abuse and eventually ends up in an institution for the deaf.

In French literature we find a deaf character in Victor Hugo's novel *'The Hunchback of Notre-Dame'* from 1831. Quasimodo is a deformed 20-year-old hunchback, who is the bell ringer of the Notre-Dame Cathedral in Paris. He is half blind and deaf, the latter as a result of all the years ringing the bells of the church. Abandoned by his mother as a baby, he was adopted by the Archdeacon Claude Frollo. Quasimodo's life takes place within the confines of the cathedral and his only two outlets are ringing the bells and express his love and devotion for Frollo. Because the citizens of Paris despise him for his appearance, he rarely ventures outside the Cathedral.

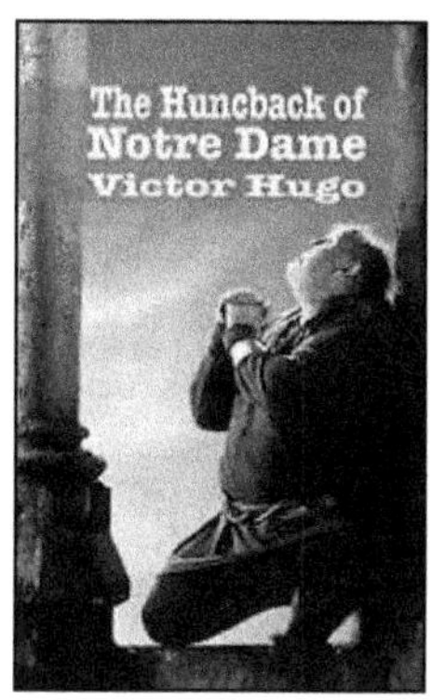

Between 1911 and 1996 the story of the hunchback was adapted for film no less than seven times, the last adaptation being an animated musical drama film, produced by the Walt Disney Animation Studios.

One of the main characters in Carson Mc Cullers' beautiful novel *'The heart is a lonely hunter'* (1943) is a deaf-mute man, Singer, who uses sign language to communicate with his best friend . We quote a small piece that reflects the spirit of the age in which the book was written (of course there were no CIs yet at that time):

> He tried to recount to himself certain things that had happened when he was young. .... Singer recalled that, although he had been deaf since he was an infant, he had not always been a real mute. He was left an orphan very young and placed in an institution for the deaf. He had learned to talk with his hands and to read. Before he was nine years old he could talk with one hand in

the American way—and also could employ both of his hands after the method of Europeans. He had learned to follow the movements of people's lips and to understand what they said. Then finally he had been taught to speak. ...

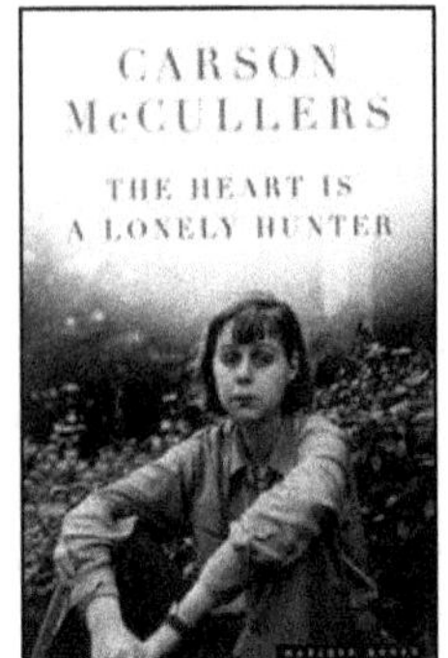

But he could never become used to speaking with his lips. It was not natural to him, and his tongue felt like a whale in his mouth....

It was painful for him to try to talk with his mouth, but his hands were always ready to shape the words he wished to say. (p. 14-15).

McCullers' book was also made into a film by Robert Ellis Miller in 1968 (see also below).

From 1875 to early 1893, Modest, the brother of composer Pyotr Tchaikovsky, took care of the deaf-mute Nikolai Germanovich Konradi, nicknamed Kolya, as a teacher and educator. He learned the child to speak. Nikolai Konradi was a son of wealthy parents and was eight years old when he came into the care of the Tchaikovsky brothers. Modest loved this boy like his own son. In the Dutch language novel *'Kolja'* the author Arthur Japin tells the story of Modest and Pyotr Ilyich Tchaikovsky, who take care of little Nikolai. They should spend seventeen years with him. Traveling through Europe they liberate the boy from his isolation. In the novel, Japin also takes a closer look at the death of Pyotr Tchaikovsky in 1893, the true cause of which is still unclear and has given rise to certain unproven speculations. The book alternates chapters from the perspective of Modest's diaries about Kolya's childhood and the speech lessons he received with chapters about Kolya's later attempts to discover the truth about Tchaikovsky's death.

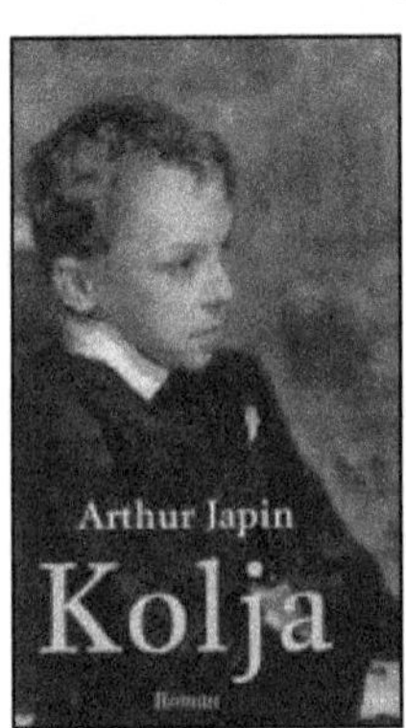

The father of the main character, Aga Akbar, in Kader Abdolah's novel *'My father's notebook'* is the deaf-mute illegitimate son of a Persian nobleman who lives in the Iranian mountains. He communicates by using a self-made sign language and he also designs his own cuneiform script to record his experiences in book form. After his death, the book ends up with his son, who fled to the Netherlands. He translates the book into legible script. This is a fascinating psychological novel about a father/son relationship, but also about love and death, loyalty and betrayal, truth and lie.

Joanne Greenberg wrote the beautiful book *'In this Sign'*, about the not obvious life of deaf people. It is the story of Abel and Janice, two young people, who leave a poorly adapted boarding school for the deaf with little or no experience. They get married and step from their protected environment into the world of the hearing. Years of poverty and labor begin, they understand nothing about the world and decide to no longer trust the hearing community. Happier times are also dawning, such as the birth of their daughter Margaret. She can hear and thus becomes the intermediary between her parents and the outside world.

Also written by Joanne Greenberg is the book *'Of such small differences'*, based on the author's work experiences with the deaf/blind. It tells the (fictional) life story of a certain John. He is twenty-six, born blind and beaten deaf by his father at the age of nine. He lives independently, has a job at a social work center and is a worthy poet. At some point, the chaotically living and impulsive actress Leda enters his life. He falls in love with her, maybe she also with him, although that is not entirely clear center and is a worthy poet. At some point, the chaotically living and impulsive actress Leda enters his life. He falls in love with her, maybe she also with him, although that is not entirely clear. He moves in

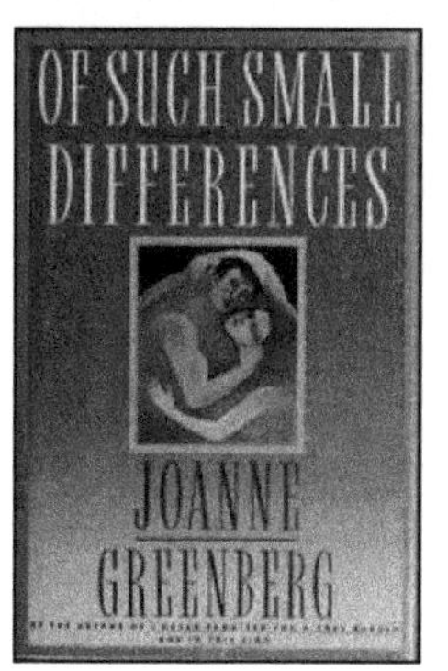

with her. Small differences gradually take on larger forms, he lives by the grace of order, and she hates monotonous regularity, a break seems inevitable. Sensitively and with great empathy, Green describes the feelings and thoughts of John, his fantasy which takes shape in his poems, which have been recorded in the book, his contacts with his own group, his frustration because of his inability to cope with seeing and hearing people, and his grief and the outbursts of anger that follow.

In the book *'Talk, talk'* by T.C. Boyle, deaf teacher Dana Halter is arrested after a minor traffic violation on suspicion of fraud and violent crime. It soon turns out that she is a victim of identity theft. After disappointing experiences with the official authorities, she decides, together with her boyfriend, to pursue the perpetrator herself. The two go on a quest across the United States, to eventually end up in Peterskill, a town not far from New York, where it comes to a violent confrontation.

In *'Deafening'* by Canadian author Frances Itani, the protagonist Grania loses her hearing due to scarlet fever and ends up in a school for the Deaf in Belleville, where she learns to sign and to speak. After finishing school, Grania meets Jim, a young hearing man with whom she falls madly in love.

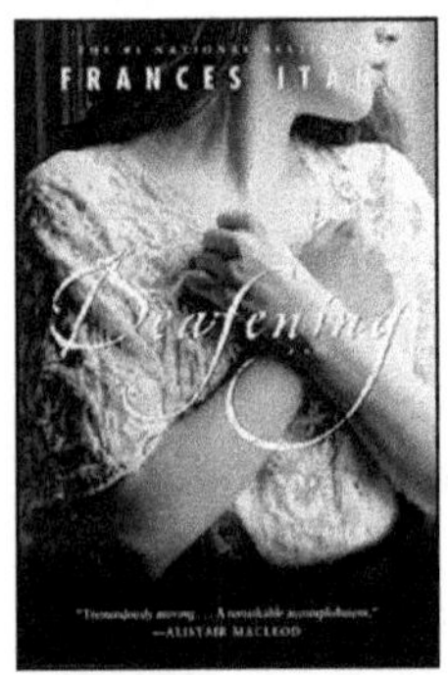

Together they discover a new language that consists of both sound and silence. Grania's life now seems to be slowing down, until World War I breaks out and the young couple is driven apart. Jim has to go to the battlefield in Flanders. Months later, traumatized, he returns to Grania, and the two question whether their love can withstand the memories of war.

Somewhat special is the book *'Resurrection Bay'* by Emma Viskic. It is an exciting thriller in which Caleb, the deaf protagonist, goes in search of the murderer of a childhood friend. But although he's now an expert in reading human expressions, misreading lips and missed words sometimes lead to confusion and trouble. The main character's deafness is what makes this book extra interesting. After all, his other senses are more developed as a result, which provides a special reading experience. It is also worth mentioning that the author has learned sign language especially for this book. She has already won several awards and nominations with this debut.

In the mystery book *'For the Sake of Elena'* (Elisabeth George, 1992) the deaf student Elena is killed whilst jogging in the morning near Cambridge college. We learn that her parents wouldn't let her learn how to sign until she was in her teens because they wanted her to live a "normal" life. Her friend from the campus Deaf Student Group despises her because she doesn't embrace Deaf culture. But who murdered her and why?

'Silent Fear' by the writing duo Lance and James Morcan is also

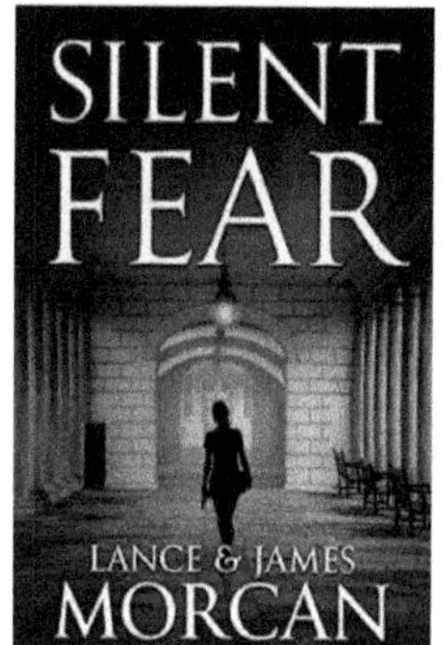

a thriller, in which Inspector Valerie Crowther is assigned to investigate the murder of a student at London's Deaf University. The murder investigation coincides with the outbreak of a deadly flu virus, which quarantines the university and thus cuts it off from the outside world. When more deaf students are subsequently murdered, it becomes clear that a serial killer is at work in the university, which is closed off from the outside world. A cat and mouse game unfolds as the killer sets his sights on Inspector Valerie and the virus kills more victims. A somewhat topical story!?

Children's books – young adult

Literature is one of the most effective ways to understand society and our place in it (Callis 2017). Children also learn through books to gain insight into relationships and conflicts and develop empathy and morality. Moreover, it teaches them to better deal with their own emotions. Callis therefore believes that books on deafness and hearing impairment should belong to any collection of children's books. Whether you are the parent of a hearing or a deaf child, in both cases confronting children with hearing difficulties can help to appreciate human diversity. She lists 10 reasons why deaf characters should appear in the books of a children's library. We adopt these below in an abridged form:

1. To teach children to understand that deafness is a medical condition with multiple degrees and forms and that persons with deafness can therefore deal with it in very different ways.
2. Teaching them to understand that there is such a thing as a Deaf culture and a Deaf identity.
3. To help children understand that sign language is a visual communication tool and why that is important.
4. Familiarize them with the characteristics of those who are deaf or hard of hearing, e.g., that they have hearing aids or CIs and sometimes talk with a "weird" accent.
5. Teaching children how to solve simple communication breakdowns in everyday situations.
6. Learning how to accept deaf and hard of hearing children as friends.
7. Teaching them the value of different groups of friends and the benefits of diversity.
8. For the deaf children to feel represented.
9. Seeing deaf and hard of hearing children as role models.
10. To see deaf and hard of hearing individuals as interesting and complex persons, worth getting to know.

In what follows we give a few examples of children's and youth books, in which (some of) the above-mentioned objectives are pursued.

Kate Gaynor wrote *'A Birthday for Ben: Children's book on Hearing Difficulties'.* Children with a hearing problem often feel different from their peers because of their hearing aids or because they can't participate in games, in which auditory stimuli are important. This story helps children to realize the difficulties such children face and how certain daily situations are frustrating for them. Deaf/hard of hearing children can learn from the main character that it is O.K. to name specific frustrations and other issues they experience. This story helps to make it clear that no child should be ignored or excluded.

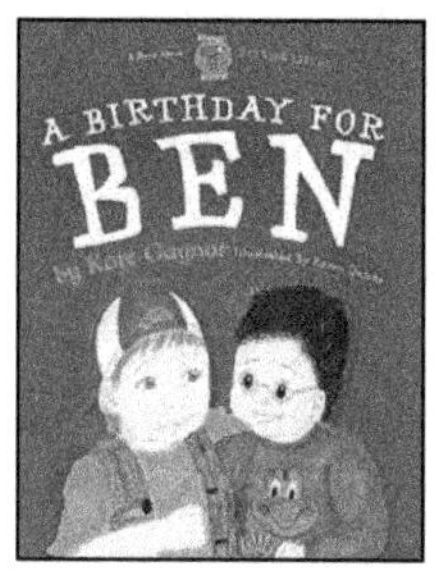

'A place for Grace' by Jean Davies Okimoto is about a little dog (Grace) with big dreams. When she discovers she is too small to be a guide dog for the blind, she runs into Charlie, a deaf man who thinks she would be a great hearing aid dog. It is a book that can help children to understand people with disabilities as well as it can offer the reader an opportunity to learn some sign language.

In Lakin and Steele's *'Dad and Me in the Morning'*, Jacob, a little deaf boy, is awakened in the morning by his special alarm clock. He puts in his hearing aids and gently wakes up his father. Together they walk to the beach and observe the surrounding nature. Father and son have a lot of ways to talk to each other: making gestures, reading lips and... just squeezing each other's hands.

'Dina the deaf dinosaur' harks back to the childhood of author Carole Addabbo, who herself is deaf from birth. The book tells the story of a young, deaf dinosaur who runs away from home because her parents do not want her to learn sign language. In the forest she befriends Otto the owl, Molière the mole and Camilla the squirrel. Fortunately, Otto knows some sign language, because he has lived underneath a deaf pigeon for a while (for children from 4 to 5 years old).

'El deafo' is a 2014 graphic novel written and illustrated by Cece Bell and intended for children and youngsters aged 8 to 12. The book is based on autobiographical elements, taken from the author's childhood and her life with a hearing impairment.

However, the characters in the book are all rabbits. Bell herself calls this ironic, because rabbits with their large ears are known for their excellent hearing. The book traces Bell's childhood, who needed hearing aids to grow up to be the person she is today. Although the hearing aids allow her to perceive the world around, they also create distance from her peers by being 'different'. This causes her frustration and depression. Eventually she comes to see her hearing aids as a 'super power' (El Deafo), because her phonic ear amplification even allows her at times to hear more than anyone else, e.g. when teachers forget to remove their microphone.

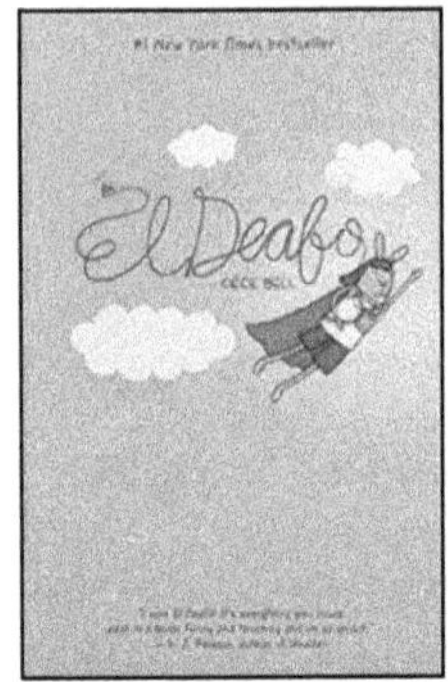

'Mila Gets Her Super Ears' is a recent book (2020), written by Ashley Machovec and illustrated by Megan Jansen. We follow Mila and her family on their journey through the world of hearing loss, hearing aids and cochlear implants. Mila herself and her family don't know what to expect. Topics like ABR[13], initial diagnosis, the listening booth, the cochlear implant procedure and the therapies that follow the implantation are described in a clear and understandable language.

In Stephanie Marrufo's book *'All the Ways I Hear You'* the young hard of hearing Sy and his neat hearing aids are first introduced. Further on, Sy introduces his diverse group of friends who are deaf, hard of hearing or deafblind.

[13] ABR: auditory brainstem response, a safe and painless test to see how the hearing nerves and brain respond to sound

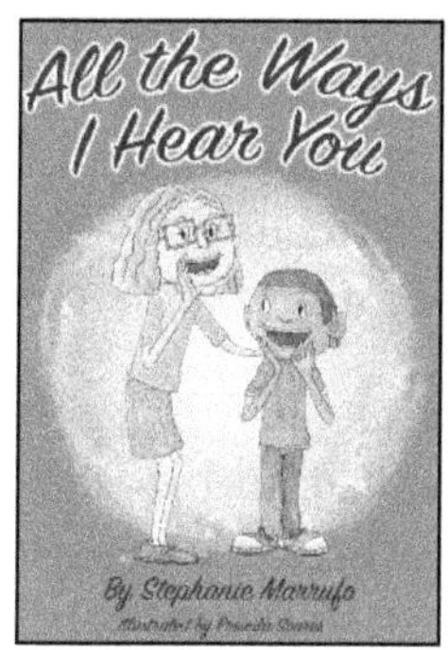

The hearing technology and communication styles they use, like cochlear implants, bone anchored hearing systems, communication boards/tablets and sign language, are described. Stephanie Marrufo, who is Sy's mom, began searching for children's books that featured or included deaf and hard of hearing characters, but she found this type of resource to be extremely lacking. That's why she wrote this book herself.

We made a very limited selection of 'young adult'-books.

In Sheryl Jordan's book *'The Raging Quiet'*, Marnie is accused of witchcraft because her new husband dies in an accident barely two days after their wedding. In the hostile environment she finds herself in, the pastor and the young Raven are the only ones willing to help her. Marnie finds out that Raven is deaf and not at all possessed by demons, as the villagers think. Together with Raven she learns to read and write and she also designs a real sign language for him, with which she once again throws oil on the witch fire. It is a fascinating story about the power of communication, but also about narrow-mindedness and intolerance. The book is intended for young adults from 13 to 15 years old

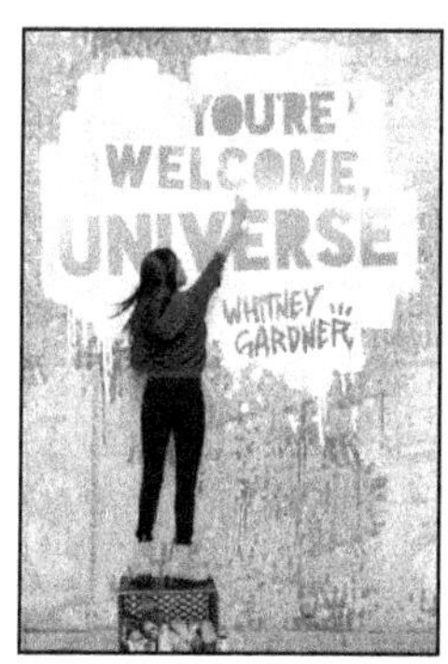

Whitney Gardner's *'You're Welcome, Universe'* is about the deaf Julia. When she sees that someone has written something insulting about her best friend on a wall of her school, she spray-paints a beautiful (and somewhat illegal) drawing over it with graffiti. She is expelled from school because of this well-intentioned action. This is a big problem for Julia, because she now has to go to another school where she will be the only deaf student. It is difficult for her to find her way at her new school. Despite a promise to her parents, Julia cannot resist continuing to make street art, challenged by an unknown person. Before she knows it, she is in the middle of a graffiti war and the police are on her heels (from 15 years).

'Of Sound Mind' by Jean Ferris has the high school senior Theo as a protagonist. He is fluent in spoken English and in sign language, because both his parents and his brother, Jeremy, are deaf. Because Theo can hear, this has made him the interpreter and go-between for his family. Things get complicated when Thomas, Theo's father, has a stroke and his mother cannot bring herself to nurse her husband, leaving Theo with the full burden to bear. But with the help of his girlfriend Ivy and some of her friends, Theo is finally able to change his family's dynamics and find time to plan his own future.

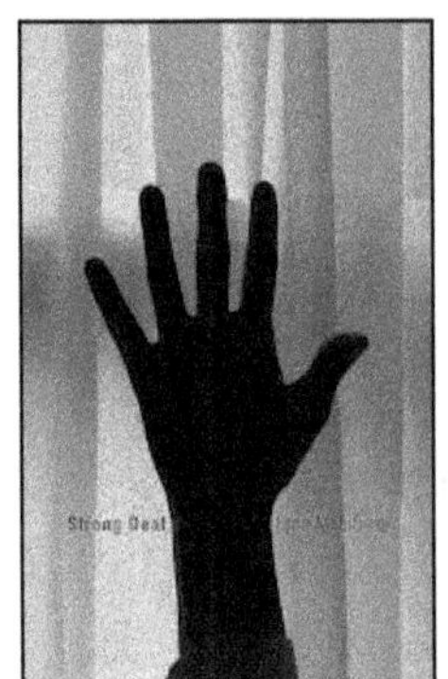

In *'Strong Deaf'*, written by Lynn E. McElfresh, Jade is the only hearing member in her family. Her siblings, parents and grandparents are deaf. Her older sister Marla lives at a school for the deaf during the week, just coming home on weekends and holidays. When they end up on the same softball team for the summer, neither is happy about it. Told from both points of view, this story gives the reader a good look inside the world of Strong Deaf and what it is like to be the outsider – in this case Jade, the only one who can hear. In spite of their differences, they finally discover that each has a lot to offer the other.

'Invisible' is a young adult book by Cecily Anne Paterson. The main character is Jazmine Crawford, who doesn't want to make decisions or to make choices and neither does she want to make friends. She only wants to be invisible. For her it's easy to take off her hearing aid and drift along pretending that nothing's wrong. Then she finally starts to come out of her

shell when she's forced to be in the school play. Invisible is a coming of age story about a young girl in Australia who is hearing impaired, whose father died when she was younger, who has no friends, a very low self-confidence, and who is being bullied at school.

Films - theater

Again we make a distinction between (semi)biographical and documentary films concerning deafness and/or hearing loss, and fiction films, in which deaf and hard of hearing characters are introduced or are part of the story.

The French documentary film *'Le Pays des sourds'* (The Land of the Deaf) was written and directed by Nicolas Philibert in 1992. In this film the question is asked how we should imagine the world of those thousands of people who live in silence. Anyone who ventures into the 'Land of the Deaf' is touched by the strange choreography of gestures that allows them to express themselves. Originated a long time ago, these gestures form a real language, in which every word and phrase is translated by an image that is formed in space. These signs are just as precise and nuanced as words and can be used for declarations of love as well as detailed technical descriptions. Jean-Claude, Abou, Philo, Hubert, Karine and all the others who appear in the film are deaf from birth and they dream, think, communicate in gestures and see the world in a different way. In this film, the viewer sets out to discover that distant, other land, where the gaze and touch are so important. This film won multiple awards between 1992 and 1997.

Another French documentary is *'J'avancerai vers toi avec les yeux d'un sourd'* (I will walk towards you with the eyes of a deaf), realized in 2014 by Laetitia Carton. This is also a film in which the characters play themselves.

The protagonists belong to different generations, but they are almost always belonging to families of deaf parents, who have deaf children. When viewing this film, one has to take the context into account. Someone born deaf in France in the 1950s-60s did not have many options. After all, since the Congress of Milan in 1880, sign language was banned and in most places only the oral method was tolerated. After all, it was assumed that (1)sign language was not a real language, (2)the word was given by God as a means of communication, and (3)gestures prevented the deaf from breathing properly and thus could provoke tuberculosis(!).

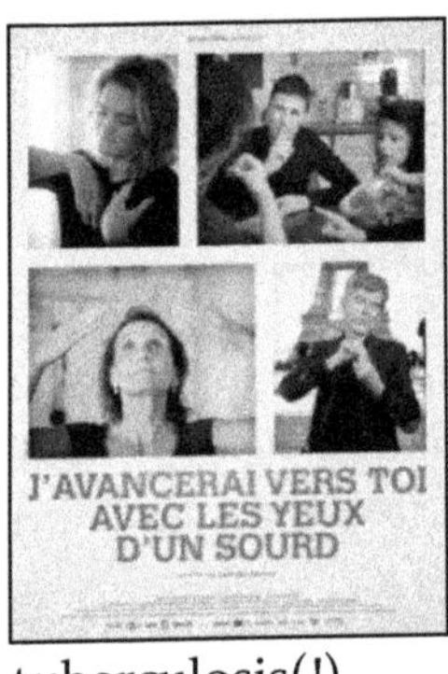

Despite this ban, sign language did not disappear and was passed on from generation to generation and used for recreation, among friends and family. It is felt that the deaf, gesticulating persons in this film are still very suspicious of "the others" and very critical of cochlear implants and towards adherents of oralism. They often don't want the medical community to "cure" their deafness in order to make them hearing.

Levent Beskardes is a deaf-born French-Turkish theater maker, poet, director, draftsman and stage designer, born in 1949. He has appeared in several films, such as the aforementioned *'Pays des Sourds'* and *'J'avancerai vers toi avec les yeux d' un sourd '*, but he also made several short films himself (Oiseau, 2000, L'Artiste, 2001, Sept péchés capitaux, 2002, Auto-film, 2003, Rêve de clown, 2004, Tremblement de Terre), in which deafness and hearing impairment are central. Beskardes also participates in the International Visual Theater, located in Paris, which is a laboratory for artistic, linguistic and pedagogical research into sign language and regarding visual and physical arts. A school for learning sign language is also located in the building.

In the U.S.A. the National Theater of the Deaf (NTD) was founded in 1967, and since then has a long and rich history as a national and even international performing arts organization. NTD pioneered a dual language theater concept, creating a hybrid of American Sign Language with spoken English.

The idea for the National Theater of the Deaf came about in the late 1950's through the Broadway production '*The Miracle Worker*', based on the true story of the deaf and blind Helen Keller (see below) and featuring actress Anne Bancroft (see also below).
Anne and David Hays, the Lighting Designer, were full of the idea of taking sign language to the stage as a performing art form. Nearly ten years later Hays succeeded to secure funding from the U.S. Department of Education to launch the National Theater of the Deaf. Since then the NTD has been seen in all fifty states in the U.S., in thirty-three other countries, and on all seven continents throughout the world. The theater has appeared and performed on Broadway, on the Disney Channel, on Sesame Street and at the White House.

An extremely illuminating documentary film is '*Through deaf eyes*', made by Lawrence Hott and Diane Garey (2007). It's a two-hour documentary exploring almost two centuries of Deaf life in the U.S.A. This film sheds light on historical facts and events that have shaped Deaf lives, but also focusses on the stories of people with hearing problems, both eminent and ordinary. Some prominent members of the Deaf community are interviewed, such as actress Marlee Matlin. Attention has been given also to the discord between adherents of oralism and supporters of Sign Language and to the pros and cons of cochlear implants. Really a must see[14]!

---

[14] See: https://www.gallaudet.edu/history-through-deaf-eyes/through-deaf-eyes-documentary

'One Deaf Child' is an interesting presentation by Rachel Coleman (2013). We also mention the documentary *'For a deaf son'*. In this film we follow Thomas, who was one year old, when his parents discovered he was profoundly deaf. His father, a filmmaker, produced the film. It tells of a family's journey as they face some life-changing decisions.

'Hear and Now' is a 2007 documentary created by Irene Taylor Brodsky, who has won awards at the Sundance Film Festival and the Heartland Film Festival as well as a Peabody Award in 2008. The filmmaker's parents were both born deaf. However, the couple had hearing children. Paul and Sally Taylor were already in their 60s when they decided to have a cochlear implant placed, which would allow them to hear for the first time. This documentary follows them in what turns out to be a very complex journey from the comfortable world of silence to the very challenging world of sound, noice and spoken language. Attention is paid to the couple's personal history, but also to the procedure itself and its aftermath. After all, the effects of the operation are not only positive.

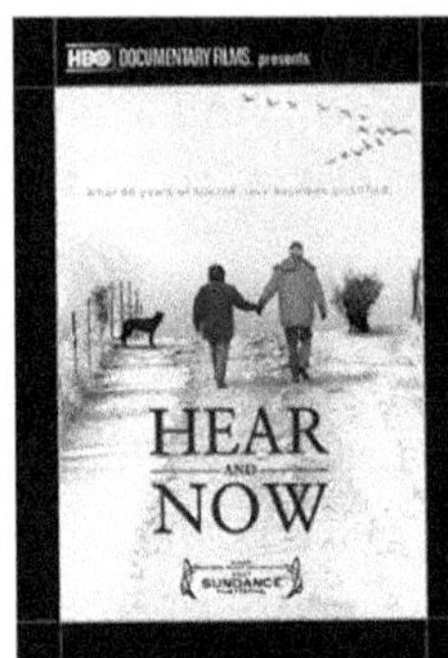

'Helen Keller in Her Story' is an American biographical documentary film about the deaf / blind Helen Keller, made in 1954 and based largely on Keller's higher mentioned autobiography. Later, in 1962, Arthur Penn made the semi-biographical film *'The Miracle Worker'* about Anne Sullivan, who was also blind herself and became Keller's teacher. The latter film met with critical acclaim and was nominated for five Oscar awards, two of which it won: best actress for Anne Bancroft (as Anne Sullivan) and best

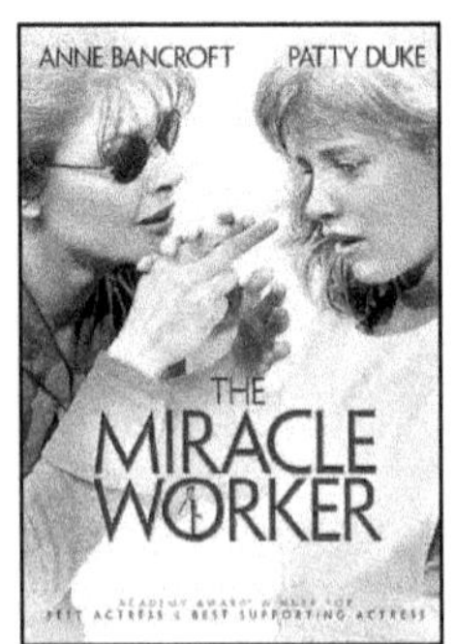

supporting actress for Patty Duke (as Helen Keller). Later, two more television adaptations were made of this film.

'Land of Silence and Darkness' (original German title: *'Land des Schweigens und der Dunkelheit'*) is a 1971 documentary film about deaf-blind people and their life experiences. The film was written, directed and produced by the famous German film producer Werner Herzog. In this film, Herzog follows Fini Straubinger, a German woman who became deaf and blind early in life, as she visits other deafblind people and comments on their struggle to survive in the modern world.

'Language Says It All' is a short American documentary film from 1987 about deaf children and their caregivers, directed by Rhyena Halpern.

'Sound and Fury' (2000) is also produced in the U.S. It is a documentary film featuring two brothers and their families. One is deaf, the other hearing. The deaf brother has a deaf wife and a deaf daughter. While the father is opposed to a CI, daughter Heather wants one. The hearing brother has a hearing wife, but the couple has a deaf baby, for whom they are considering the possibilities of a CI. The film explores the not always evident relationship between the Deaf community and cochlear implantation. In the follow-up documentary *'Sound and Fury: 6 Years Later'* (2006), Heather is twelve years old and she, her two sisters, her mother and other relatives of her deaf family all eventually opted for a CI. She now appears to have clear speech, to live in the "normal" world, to interact with hearing people and to achieve good grades in school. Heather moves smoothly in the world of both hearing and deaf, and she embraces the Deaf culture just as she has hearing friends. She is currently in her twenties.

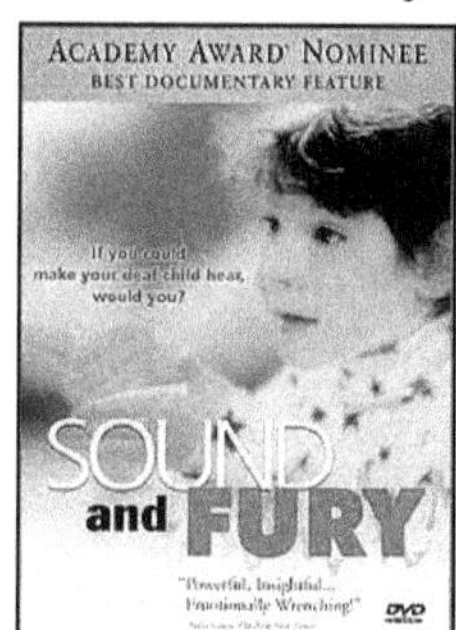

On the internet many other short films and documentaries on deafness, hearing loss and Deaf culture can be found. It would lead us too far to describe them all.

With regard to fiction films, Lerner (2010) describes that films, in which deaf characters appear, often do not focus at all on the condition of deafness. Rather, they seem to play a role in advancing the plot of the story or give a better understanding of hearing people in the film (see also Dakin's earlier comment, 2009). The deaf persons can play a symbolic role, for example as a metaphor for the isolation felt by those who have no voice in society. Misunderstanding auditory stimuli can sometimes give rise to comical situations or can sometimes rescue them from a predicament. Due to its unique linguistic properties and the fact that hearing people do not understand it, sign language can in some cases bring salvation to a storyline. Deaf people are shown in films in different domains and in different countries. Films thus influence and reflect cultural attitudes and views and can especially have an important influence on hearing people who have had little or no contact with the world of the deaf and the hard of hearing. Lerner went through a number of search engines to find as many films as possible, in which people with deafness or hearing loss appeared. She did not distinguish whether or not the actors were really deaf or hard of hearing - something that is a delicate issue in the Deaf community - and came to the following classification:

- Deafness as part of the plot
- Deaf persons as informants of the protagonist
- Deaf characters as a parallel to the protagonist
- Sign language as the "hero" of the story
- Stories with relationships between the deaf and the hearing
- An ordinary boy or girl who happens to be deaf
- Deafness as a psychosomatic consequence of trauma

- Deafness as a metaphor

- Deafness as a symbolic commentary on society

- Let the hands speak

In what follows, we will briefly review each of these categories.

In a first category, deafness is an essential part of the plot. Every element of a movie is basically a means of developing the plot, but if the story centers around a character who is deaf, its success depends on a particular person displaying a particular condition, in this case, deafness. The limitations or advantages of the deaf person functioning in the hearing world determine the tension, comedy or other events that make up the story (Lerner, 2010). For example, in the film *'Hear no Evil'* (see also below) the deaf Jillian learns which noise-making things cause her hearing friend a splitting headache: she activates the smoke alarm when toasting toast, she throws a metal spoon in the iron garbage can with a lot of noise....
Another example of such a film is Peter Yates' 1987 *'Suspect'*, in which Liam Neeson plays a deaf, homeless Vietnam veteran who is unfairly accused of murder. Advocate Cher defends him and exposes the truth. The film *'Read my lips'* (French title: Sur mes Lèvres) also belongs in this category (discussion, see below).

'The sound of metal' is a recent film (2019, directed by Darius Marder) starring Riz Ahmed as a metal drummer who loses his hearing. First he tries to learn American Sign Language, later he sells his drums and other music equipment, using the money for cochlear implant surgery. When the implants are activated, he is very disappointed by their distorted sound.
This film got six nominations at the 2021 Academy Awards and won two of them (Best Sound and Best Film Editing).

The potentially comical aspects of deafness may seem very politically incorrect nowadays. Although often innocent and not intended to harm the deaf population, the deafness acts as a kind of banana peel over which the characters stumble. An example of this is the 1989 film *'See no evil, hear no evil'*, in which Gene Wilder and Richard Pryor portray a deaf and a blind person respectively. The film is a sequence of jokes and misunderstandings that arise as a result of lip reading and blindness.

Robert Moore's (1976) comedy *'Murder by death'* revolves around a dinner invitation to five world-famous detectives to solve a murder case. The sender is Lionel Twain, an eccentric millionaire who lives in a lonely, gloomy mansion with a sinister, blind butler and a deaf-mute cook.

In a second category, the deaf persons act as informants of the protagonists. Their first function is to provide the audience with more information about the hearing characters or to generate more affinity with them. The deaf person may be fascinating in and of him/her self, but in general, the hearing impairment is only marginally important. The audience's attitude towards the hearing characters is influenced by their past or current involvement with deaf individuals. We give two examples of films from this category. In the 1992 movie *Gas, Food, Lodging'* directed by Allison Anders, a certain Shade discovers that bad boy Javier's mother is deaf. Javier introduces Shade to his mother through simple gestures and fingerspelling. They go out together and they dance (the mother feels the vibrations on the floor). He movie audience is led to sympathize with Javier: "he's a soft soul in a rough shell, because look how sensitive he grew up with an exotic, deaf mother".

The movie *'Looking for Mrs Goodbar'* (1977) confronts movie lovers with Theresa (role played by Diane Keaton), a somewhat confused young woman who leads a double life. By day she is a dedicated teacher for the deaf, but at night she frequents shady bars and indulges in sexual exploits. The film shows how with her early use of gestures she begins to express her deepest desires as well as her ability to communicate and connect with her students.

Other films in which deaf characters are introduced in support of the hearing are *'Miracle on 34th Street'* (1994 version), *'Nashville'* (1975, directed by Robert Altman), *'The Family Stone'* (2005, directed by Thomas Bezucha), *'Grand Canyon'* (1991, directed by Lawrence Kasdan) and *'There Will Be Blood'* by Paul Thomas (2007). In the last mentioned, the adopted son of the main character (role of Daniel Day-Lewis) becomes deaf as a result of a gas explosion.

In the third category, which Lerner distinguishes, there are two parallel storylines, one with a hearing character and one with a deaf person. A good example is *'I Don't Want to Talk about It*, a 1993 Argentinian film directed by María Luisa Bemberg. In this we see Charlotte, a girl with dwarfism, who befriends with Reanalde, who is deaf. Both mothers sympathize and although the story is mainly about Charlotte, the parallel line about the deaf girl remains in the background. The story takes place in the 1930s and the viewer can assume that awareness of disabilities was still very minimal back then. Although Charlotte's counterpart is little in the picture, it is clear that both girls must fight a similar struggle for recognition and acceptance.

In the fourth category, sign language plays a role as a hero and even as a lifesaver. The best example of this is the 1994 film *'The River Wild'* by director Curtis Hanson and starring Meryl Streep as Gail Hartman. Gail is familiar with sign language because her father is deaf. Mother, father and son are therefore able to communicate with each other secretly and subtly through gestures behind the back of a bunch of criminals and thus are able to escape from a predicament.

The fifth category concerns relationships between deaf and hearing persons. Of course, with the increased awareness and acceptance of deafness, it is tempting to think that a relationship with a deaf person is not in itself too much of a challenge. More subtitles, more sign language interpreters, more inclusion in education lead to better integration and greater visibility in the public domain. Nevertheless, a number of important issues remain underexposed, such as the opposing views on the pedagogical approach of the deaf and dealing with family members and peers who speak a “different” language.

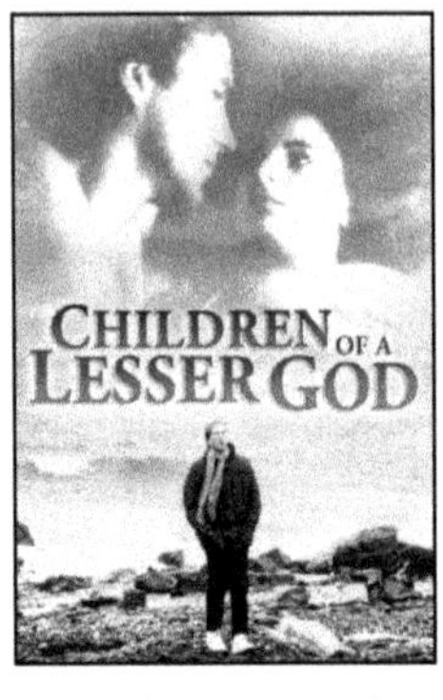

The 1986 American drama *'Children of a lesser God'* directed by Randa Haines, shows an example of a relationship between the deaf Sarah and the hearing James and the resulting controversies. The film is based on the 1980 play of the same name by American author Mark Medoff. The new teacher at a school for the deaf falls in love with Sarah, the deaf janitor, a very intelligent young woman, who, however, has completely cut herself off from everything and everyone. At the heart of their struggle is James's inability to accept that Sarah is complete the way she is, as a nonspeaking, but signing, deaf woman. The highly esteemed deaf teacher must accept for himself that he can learn much from her. William Hurt is heartwarming as James, the deaf actress Marlee Matlin is very convincing in the role of Sarah. Matlin won the Academy Award for Best Actress and the Golden Globe for Best Actress in a drama movie for her performance. As stated earlier, Medoff's play was also translated in French and put on the stage with a splendid Emmanuelle Laborit in the leading role.

Another movie in this category is *'Johnny Belinda'* originally from 1949, but which was made a TV movie starring Mia Farrow in 1967 and later, in 1982, got another television adaptation. This film tells the harrowing story of the deaf and mute girl Belinda. When a new family doctor settles on Cape Breton Island, where she lives, he soon discovers that Belinda is very sensible and he wants to teach her how to read lips. However, she is later raped by the local bully Locky McCormick and becomes pregnant. The villagers believe that Belinda will not be a suitable mother and the child is assigned to the rapist.

Robert Markowitz's 1979 film *'Voices'* is about a young deaf woman, Rosemarie, who is a deaf teacher and whose big dream it is to become a dancer, something her mother does not support at all. Drew is a hearing truck driver who dreams of becoming a singer and who is laughed at by his brother and his father. The two meet and their relationship is made stronger by the need for support, which they both share. Other movies in this category include *Mr. Holland's Opus'* by Stephen Herek from 1995, about a music teacher and composer who has a deaf son, *'Jenseits der Stille'* '(Eng.: Beyond Silence) from 1996 by Caroline Link about a hearing daughter with deaf parents, and *'The Good Shepherd'*, a more recent film (2006) directed by Robert De Niro. In this film, the protagonist (Matt Damon) has a relationship with a deaf woman who can read lips. The very beautiful 1999 film *'Compensation'* deals with two parallel love stories, one in 1900 and one in 1990, both between a black deaf woman and a black hearing man.

The best way to measure equality is to be accepted for your own merits, regardless of any consideration for differences or limitations. Lerner calls this category 'an ordinary boy or girl, who also happens to be deaf'. A good example is *'Crazy Moon'*, a 1987 film by Allan Eastman. In this film, Brooks is a shy, eccentric young, hearing man who urgently needs to get his life back on track. He meets Vanessa, who is deaf and works as a shop assistant, while also taking speech lessons. She has an incredible "joie de vivre" that Brooks admires and wants to emulate. When one looks at the way they both interact with the world, it is clear that not Vanessa, but Brooks is the one with limitations.

In *'Requiem for a dream'*, a film by Darren Aronofsky (2000), the protagonist meets a deaf drug dealer, who speaks but also uses sign language.

Only in very exceptional cases can deafness develop as a result of a post-traumatic stress disorder, but this is of course an attractive alternative for filmmakers. In the rock musical and movie *"Tommy"*, with the music by the Who, the hero is a deaf-mute and blind boy. He went deaf when he saw his father murdered by his stepfather, a murder in which his mother was an accomplice. Growing up, he develops inner vision and discovers himself.

Hearing loss is sometimes presented as a metaphor and personification of isolation, and/or helplessness, because the general public (wrongly) assumes that those who are deaf are veiled in complete silence and in an inability to say anything. In the aforementioned movie *'Mr. Holland's Opus'* (1995), the music-loving father assumes that his deaf son will not only be unable to share his passion for music, but is also capable of little or nothing for the rest. He is condescending about the boy's dreams, so that the distance between the two keeps growing. Other films in this category are *'Rambling Rose'* with Laura Dern from 1991 (directed by Martha Coolidge), *'Babel'* (2006, directed by Alejandro González Iñárritu), featuring a deaf Japanese teenage girl, the aforementioned adaptation of the book *'The Heart Is a Lonely Hunter* '(1968, directed by Robert Ellis Miller) and the French-Romanian film *'Code inconnu* '(English title' A Code Unknown ', 2000), in which one of the characters is a teacher of the deaf and his little sister one of his students.

The penultimate category presents deafness as a symbolic commentary on society. This gives a picture of how people viewed deafness and hearing impairment in different countries, cultures and time periods. An example of this is the Chinese masterpiece *'To Live'* (1994, directed by Zhang Yimou). When the main character returns home after a captivity, his daughter turns out to have become partially deaf and mute due to a fever attack. The film cites historical and political reasons why the girl became deaf. Later on, the lack of qualified doctors will lead to her death.

'Illtown' from 1998 stars a couple of drug dealers who take care about the deaf brother of a man who has run away from home.

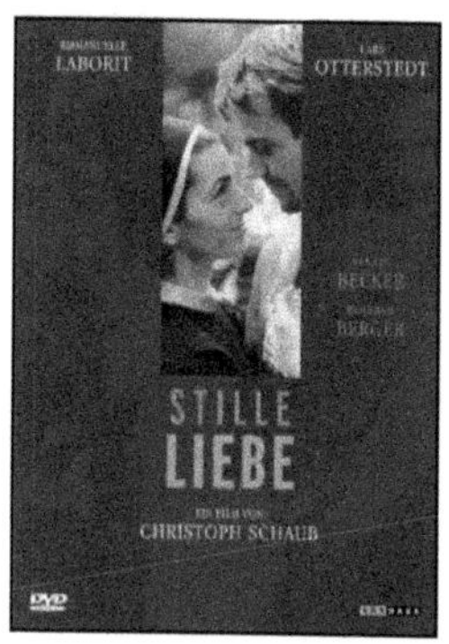

'Stille Liebe' (Quiet Love), a Swiss film from 2001 by Christoph Schaub, is featuring a 28-year-old, deaf-mute lay sister Antonia from a nunnery near the city of Zurich (role of the aforementioned, deaf actress Emmanuelle Laborit). During the day she does social work in the kitchen of a homeless shelter. Here she meets Mikas (Otterstedt), an illegal immigrant from Latvia, who, like her, is deaf. He tells her (in sign language) that he is a circus performer and is in transit. In reality he is a pickpocket who is wanted by the police and he can count on an expulsion.

The French film *'Ridicule'* (Ridiculous, directed by Patrice Leconte, 1996) is set in the 18th century and revolves around a number of hearing aristrocrats, who try to ridicule each other. If they try to do the same with a group of deaf people, they are given tit for tat.

In the feature film *'In the Company of Men'* (directed by Neil LaBute, 1997), two businessmen, Chad and Howard, are passed over for a promotion and dumped by their girlfriend. Moreover, they are both placed at a branch of the company far outside civilization for 6 weeks. Chad thinks he knows a way to make them both feel better and more confident. In order to take revenge on the female half of humanity, they decide to find a very vulnerable woman to get into her head and then drop her hard. They set their eyes on Christine, a deaf employee.

The last category Lerner mentions is: let the hands speak. In this type of film, sign language is used by a deaf character to express something that a hearing person cannot (or does not want to) convey. It is a smart tool that uses silent language to establish a communication symbiosis: someone asks a hearing person, who knows sign language, what the deaf person just said and the hearing person must express what he or she really feels but has difficulty to express him or herself. The 1996 film *'Jerry Maguire'* (directed by Cameron Crowe) stars Tom Cruise as Jerry and Renée Zellweger as Dorothy. When a deaf couple in love steps into the elevator with them, Dorothy translates the man's gestures as "You make me perfect," a strong feeling. Later, Jerry repeats this phrase exactly the same, meaning this from the bottom of his heart.

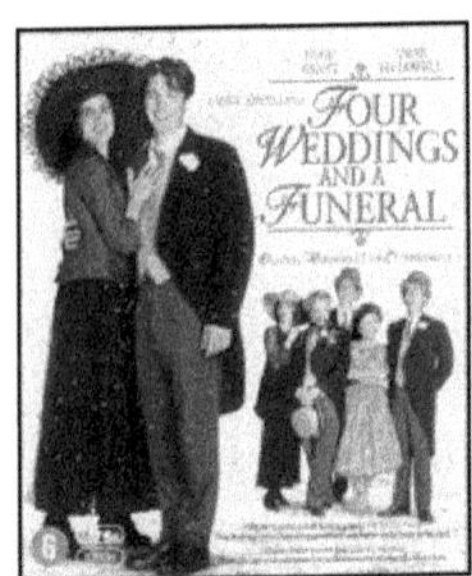

In *'Four Weddings and a Funeral'* (1994), directed by Mike Newell, actor David Bower, who is a Theater of the Deaf graduate himself, plays the deaf-mute brother of the protagonist Charles (Hugh Grant). At Charles's wedding, the churchgoers are given the opportunity to object to the marriage ("or remain silent forever"). David demands attention, requiring Charles to translate his sign language. David says he thinks the wedding should not take place because the groom loves someone else. Charles confesses that this is indeed the case, with all its consequences.

In what follows we will go through a few more films, in which deafness and/or hearing loss play an important role, without them explicitly fitting into one of the above-described categories or to be classified in several categories.

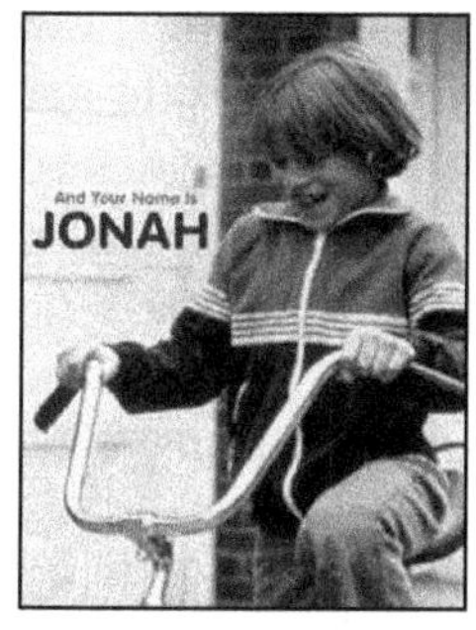

A beautiful, classic film about deafness is '*... And Your Name Is Jonah*' from 1979 (director: Richard Michaels). The lead role is played by a deaf boy, Jeffrey Bravin. This film is considered by many to be a turning point in the acceptance of deaf actors, where previously the roles of persons with deafness were played by hearing people. In the movie, Jonah is a lonely, deaf child who has been misdiagnosed as mentally retarded. We follow him in his voyage of discovery as a deaf person, from the moment he leaves the institution for retarded children to the moment he learns to communicate. Jonah's mother (Sally Struthers) and father (James Woods) try to communicate with their withdrawn child and eventually succeed through sign language. The key scene of the film is the one in which Jonah discovers that he can express himself with gestures[15]. This scene has sometimes been compared to the scene from '*The Miracle Worker*', where Helen Keller first understands what "language" is.

'*Amy*' is a 1981 film from the Walt Disney Studios. In 1913, Amy Medford (Jenny Agutter), a young mother who recently lost her beloved deaf son, leaves her wealthy, possessive husband to start a new life as a deaf teacher in a school for deaf and blind children. Although she is opposed by some people who think it is impossible to teach the deaf to speak, she persists. By helping her students overcome their limitations, she also learns to become self-reliant and independent of her husband.

'*La famille Belier*' (The Belier Family) is a 2014 French feel-good movie from director Eric Lartigau. Everyone in the Bélier family is deaf except for 16-year-old Paula. She is the indispensable interpreter in her parents' daily life, especially when it comes to the family farm.

---

[15] See for this scene: https://www.youtube.com/watch?v=WTHkfYz7hus

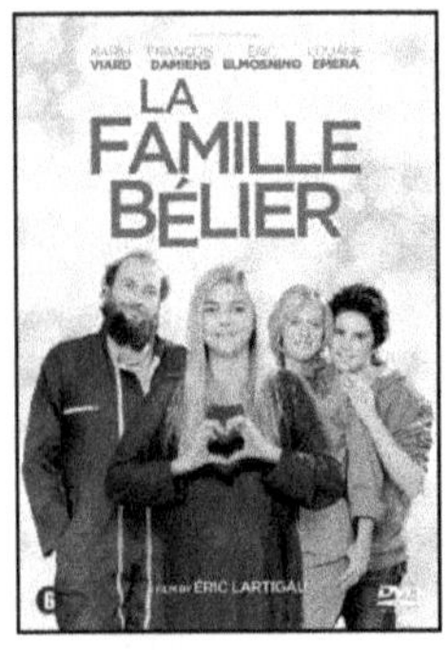

Her music teacher, Monsieur Tomasson, discovers her musical gift and encourages her to sing. Afterwards, Paula decides to take part in a prestigious singing competition in Paris for the 'Maîtrise de Radio France', the choral school of the French public broadcaster. However, that decision means leaving her family to take her first steps towards independence and adulthood.

A 1996 film by Alan Rosenberg is *'After the silence'*. Laura is a neglected deaf girl of 14 years old who has never learned sign language. A social worker takes care of her.

The movie *'Bridge to silence'* was directed by Karen Arthur (1989). Lee Remick and again Marlee Matlin are starring. John and Peg are both deaf and have a six-year-old daughter, Lisa. On their way to Peg's parents they have a car accident in which John dies. Peg has a nervous breakdown and her mother temporarily takes care of Lisa. But when Peg recovers, her mother refuses to relinquish the care of Lisa and files a lawsuit to be appointed as the child's guardian.

In the 1983 film *'Tin man'* directed by John Thomas, a young man born deaf invents a computer that allows him to hear and speak to others.

*'Sur mes lèvres (*To my lips*)* is a 2001 film by Jacques Audiard. Carla, a young woman who has hearing aids, works as a low-paid secretary at a real estate agency. Her sad and lonely life takes a different turn when 25-year-old Paul comes to work there, after serving a prison sentence. A romance develops between the two.

'Dead Silence' is a 1997 TV movie based on Jeffrey Deaver's novel *'A Maiden's Grave'* and starring James Garner. The plot of the book and movie is based on a true incident in which a

group of eight deaf students and their two teachers are held hostage by three escaped criminals. Marlee Matlin also plays a role in this film, as in the already aforementioned *'Hear no evil'*, a 1993 film by Robert Greenwald, in which she plays alongside Martin Sheen. We give the brief content of this film: Jillian Shanahan is a deaf woman and fitness trainer who is unaware that one of her clients, journalist Mickey O'Malley, has hidden a rare stolen coin in her pager. They both become the target of an unscrupulous and corrupt cop who wants the coin for himself. After Mickey's car was blown up and he dies, the cop comes after her.

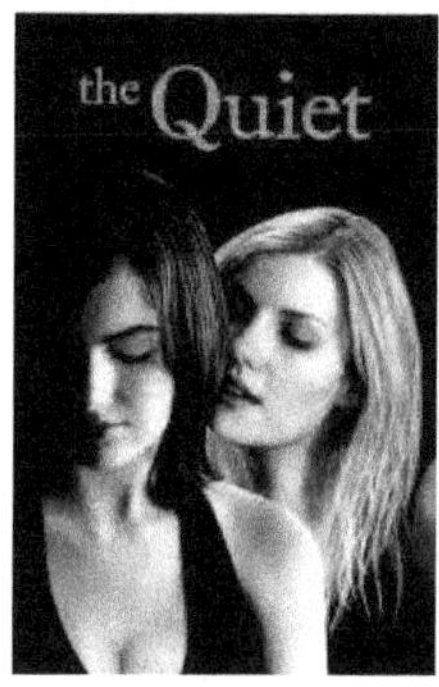

We find simulated deafness in two films. *'The Quiet'* is an American drama and thriller from 2005. The film is about the deaf-mute girl Dot, who lost her mother due to cancer at a young age and who, after her also deaf-mute father was run over by a truck, is taken into the home of her godparents Paul and Olivia Deer and their daughter Nina. The latter does not like Dot and constantly teases her. Father Paul and daughter Nina turn out to have an incestuous relationship. Then Nina discovers that Dot is not at all deaf and mute, but she does not show this. She tells Dot that she plans to kill her father, knowing that she can understand her.

Another case of simulated deafness can be found in Milos Forman's well-known 1975 film *'One Flew Over the Cuckoo's Nest'*, starring a grandiose Jack Nicholson as McMurphy. The film is based on the higher mentioned book by Ken Kesey from 1962 with the same title. Later, in 1990, the book was also turned into a theater adaptation. One of the characters is Chief Bromden, who everyone thinks is deaf and mute. When McMurphy finally provokes him, he realizes the reason for this sham. After all, Chief states: "It wasn't me who started pretending to be deaf, it were the others who started pretending I was too stupid to hear, see or say anything.

References chapter 6

Abdolah, K. (2007). *My Father's Notebook.* Harper Perennial, New York.

Addabbo, C. (2005) *Dina the deaf dinosaur.* Hannacroix Creek Books, Buchanan.

Bell, C. (2014). *El deafo.* Abrams books, New York.

Blume, S. (2006). *Grenzen aan genezen. Over wetenschap, technologie en de doofheid van een kind.* Uitgever Bert Bakker, Amsterdam.

Bollag, F., Hummel P., Kuepper A., van Beusekom R. (2006). *Das Mädchen, das aus der Stille kam*, Ehrenwirth Verlag, Mûnchen.

Boyle, TC. (2006). *Talk, talk.* Viking Press, New York.

Callis, L. (2017). *Discovering Deafness Through Children's Literature.* Retrieved 08/03/2020, from https://www.huffpost.com/entry/discovering-deafness-thro_b_14329102

Collins, W. (1854). *Hide and seek.* Richard Bentley, London.

Dakin, P. (2009). Literary portrayals of deafness. *Clinical Medicine*, 9; 293-294.

Davies Okimoto, G. (1996). *A place for Grace.* Sasquatch Books, Seattle.

Drolsbaugh, M. (1997). *Deaf Again.* Handwave Publications, Spring House.

Drolsbaugh, M. (2004). *'Anything But Silent'.* Handwave Publications, Spring House.

Ferris, J. (2004). *Of sound mind.* Farrar, Straus and Giroux, New York.

Gardner, W. (2017). *You're welcome, universe.* Knopf, New York.

Gaynor, K. (2009). *A Birthday for Ben: Children's book on Hearing Difficulties.* Special stories Publishing, Dublin.

George, E. (1992). *For the Sake of Elena, Bantam books,* New York.

Girma, H. (2000). *Haben: The Deafblind Woman Who Conquered Harvard Law,* Twelve, New York.

Greenberg, J. (1984). *In this sign*. Holt Paperbacks, Cromer.
Greenberg, J. (1989). *Of such small differences*. Signet Book, New York.
Hammond, M. (2016) *What Did You Say?: An Unexpected Journey Into the World of Hearing Loss*. Two Harbors Press, Minneapolis.
Hugo, V. (1831). *Notre-Dame de Paris*. Gosselin, Paris.
Hugo, V. (2001). *The Hunchback of Notre-Dame*. Signet Classics, New York.
Itani, F. (2003). *Deafening*. HarperCollins Canada, Toronto.
Japin, A. (2017). *Kolja*. De Arbeiderspers, Amsterdam.
Jordan, S. (2004). *The Raging Quiet'*. Simon Pulse, New York.
Laborit, E. (1999). *The Cry of the Gull,* Gallaudet University Press, Washington.
Lakin,P., Steele, R. (1994). *Dad and me in the morning*. Albert Whitman & Company, Park Ridge, Illinois.
Lerner, M.N. (2010).Narrative Function of Deafness and Deaf Characters in Film. *M/C Journal (Journal of Media and Culture)*, Vol 13, No 3.
Machovec, A, (ill. Jansen, M.)(2020). *Mila Gets Her Super Ears.* Independently published.
Marrufo, S. (2019). *All the Ways I Hear You.* Stephanie Marrufo Books, s.l.
McCullers, C. (1943. *The heart is a lonely hunter*. Houghton Mifflin, Boston.
McElfresh, L.E. (2012). *Strong Deaf.* Namelos, s.l.
Moran, L.& J. (2017). *Silent Fear*. Sterling Gate Books Ltd, s.l.
Myers, D. (2000). *A Quiet World: Living with Hearing Loss*. Yale University Press, New Haven.
Paterson, C.A. (2015). *Invisible*. Published by Cecily Paterson, s.l.
Posthuma, E. (2009). *Cochleaire capriolen. Gehoor in beweging*. Elikser, Leeuwarden.
Rodriguez, M. (2012). *Hear Your Life: Inspiring Stories and Honest Advice for Overcoming Hearing Loss*. Greenleaf Book Group Press, Austin Texas.

Sacks, O. (1989). *Seeing voices.* University of California Press, Berkeley.

Sidransky, R. (2006). *In silence. Growing up hearing in a deaf world*. Gallaudet University Press, Washington.

Silver, R. (2012). *Invisible. My Journey Through Vision and Hearing Loss.* iUniverse, Bloomington.

Spradley, S., Spradley, J. (1985). *Deaf like me.* Gallaudet University Press, Washington.

Viskic, E. (2019). *Resurrection bay*. Pushkin Vertigo, London.

Yearsley, M. (1925). Deafness in literature. *The Lancet,* 205 (5301); 746-748.

Chapter 7: Other speech and language problems

In this last chapter we bring together some speech and language problems, that are less common in books, movies or other popular media. We will successively discuss cleft lip and palate, voice problems and developmental speech and language disorders.

Cleft palate

Cleft palate (CP) is a collective term for cleft lips, jaw and palate. This is a fairly common congenital facial defect (about 1/750 births). The condition can be idiopathic, but is often part of a genetic syndrome (Kummer, 2008). Cleft palate is usually accompanied by more or less serious speech disorders, such as pronunciation problems and hypernasality.

In the visual arts there are many representations of people with clefts in the lips, jaw and/or palate (Saman, Gross, Ovchinsky & Wood-Smith, 2012). The way in which persons with CP are portrayed in sculptures and in paintings reflects the social attitudes and beliefs that people had in different time periods towards people with facial abnormalities. Very often these people were and are still being stigmatized and presented negatively. Their disturbed speech often magnifies this negative image.

Real stories from people living with cleft lip and palate can be found on the following websites:

https://www.cdc.gov/ncbddd/birthdefects/stories/cleftlip.html

https://bwc.nhs.uk/cleft-patient-stories/

https://www.cleftsmile.org/smile-stories/

Let's first give some examples of **children's books** on cleft lip and palate.

'Zoe, A Cool Cleft Kid' by Beth Gore (2011) is a non-fiction children's book about a child who has a cleft lip and palate. This book explores the medical, social and emotional aspects a cleft affected child typically faces. A photographic view of Zoe's experiences gives readers an insider's look into the world of cleft. We follow Zoe's journey through surgeries, cruel words and just wanting to let people know she is just a "regular" kid, who happens to have a cleft due to Goldenhar Syndrome. Lots of pictures accompany the simple text..

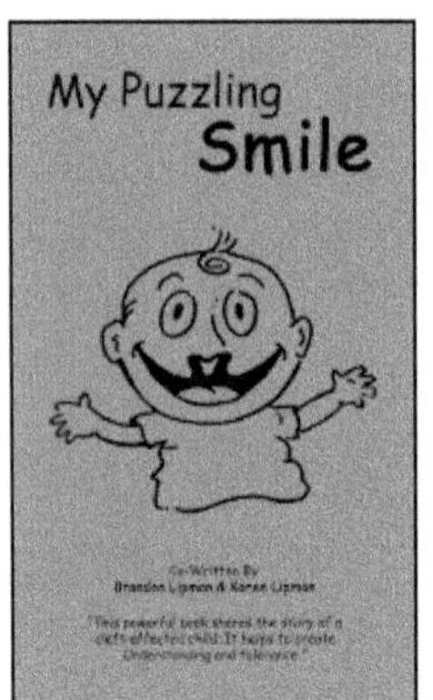

Bradon Lipman's first published book is titled *'My Puzzling Smile'*. Born with a cleft palate, the book outlines the young author's experience with being different. With the assistance of his mother, Brandon wrote his book when he was in kindergarten to explain to his classmates that his physical appearance didn't make him more different than anybody else.

'Jack's New Smile: Having a baby with cleft lip and palate' is written by Ruth Trivelpiece, Suzanne West, Jennifer Rhodes and Brooke Nunez. It is addressed to brothers and sisters of a new baby with cleft lip/palate. Baby Jack's experiences with cleft lip and palate are recounted through the eyes of his older sister. The book is also intended for children born with a cleft to help them learn about themselves. It is also meant to provide some answers to questions children may not know how or dare to ask. By reading this story, a CP child will hopefully know that having a cleft doesn't need to be scary or bad. The book can also be used as a starting point for a more detailed talk with older children. The book is also available in Spanish under the title *'La Nueva Sonrisa de Jack'*.

'Beth and her Cleft' by Nicholas Bastidas and Natalia Scabuso is an illustrated children's book designed to help children, their siblings, and their families understand all about cleft lip and palate. It is written through the eyes of an older sibling who

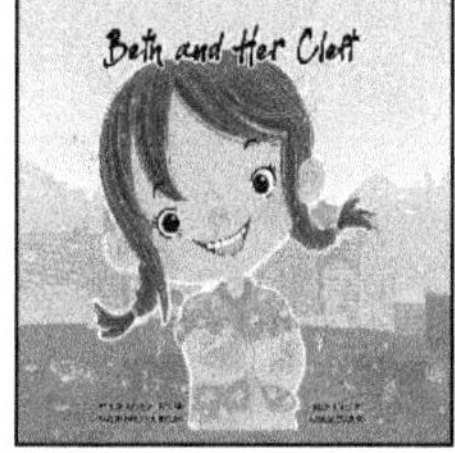

was first confused about why her baby sister looked and spoke differently. She observes her sisters progression through the necessary surgeries and supportive steps taken to treat Beth's cleft lip and palate. The love and support of her family help Beth to become confident and strong. The book is written in rhyming verses and is easy for children to follow. The author is a pediatric plastic and craniofacial surgeon based in New York. He wrote this book to help families speak openly about clefts and to comprehend the timeline and events required to treat cleft lip and palate.

'Cleft Talk for Kids', by Melissa Johnston-Burnham is an informative and interactive book that explains the condition of cleft lip and palate in a child-friendly format. In this book children and their caregivers meet Kate and Charlie, best friends who were born with clefts. Kate and Charlie explain to young readers why clefts happen and how having a cleft can affect someone on a daily basis. They also share how children with clefts are similar to their peers despite some physical difference.

Belgian Mariette Vermeylen-Nuyts is herself the mother of a

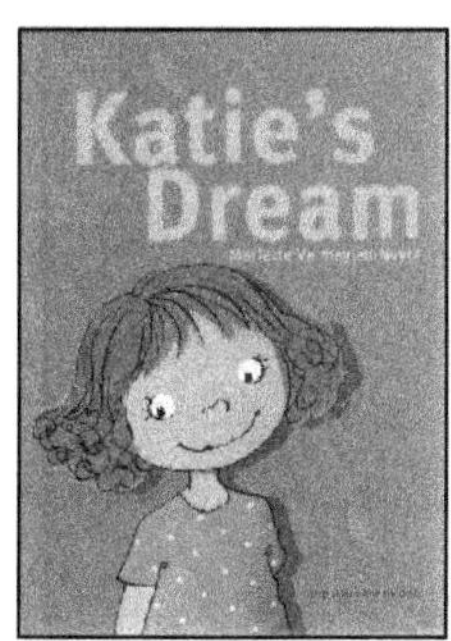

child with a cleft problem and a facial defect. She looked for information, both for parents and for children with this condition. However, she couldn't find many children's book on this topic and so decided to write one herself, entitled *'Katie's dream'* (original Dutch title: 'De droom van Kaat). In the book Katie would like to learn to play the flute, but due to her lip and palate cleft it is more of a challenge than she had hoped. With the help of a boyfriend, she visits other children in the world who do play all kinds of instruments, despite their cleft problem. For the time being she decides to learn to play another instrument until her palate has been operated completely and she might be able to learn to play the flute after all. Recommended for children from 6 years on.

In *'Smile With Simon'* by Patricia Ann Simon, Simon is a bright, red cardinal, hatched from his shell with a big gap in his beak. The gap made it hard for him to eat. Simon was not strong enough to fly. One day, he accidentally fell out of the nest and couldn't get back to his family. Patty discovered the little bird and realized he suffered from the same thing as she did, being a cleft lip. A story of friendship, love, acceptance, and kindness, this playful picture book for children shares the importance a smile has on others. It teaches a powerful lesson: despite people's differences, we are alike and beautiful.

The children's book *'First Place'* by Kate Gaynor (2007) is intended to help children realize that there are more children who suffer from similar speech problems. The main character teaches the children that they can overcome their problem by cooperating well with the speech therapist and not being afraid to keep trying. The booklet also gives parents an opportunity to talk to their children about the feelings and fears they have because of their speech difficulties. The story concerns a girl with a cleft problem, but it can also be used for children with other speech problems.

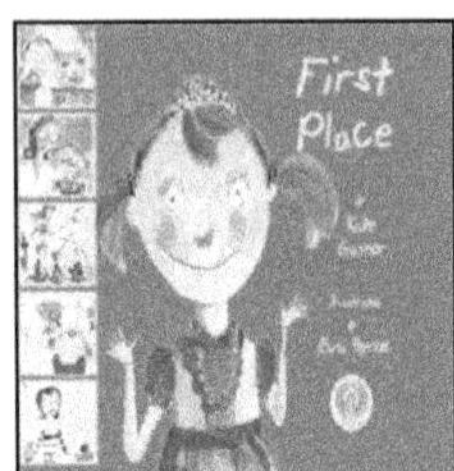

Julie Graham's *'A Special Smile'* (2006) aims to be a resource for parents, teachers and friends of children, who are different because of their "special smile". It is explained in simple words what a cleft lip and palate are. It can also be used as a tool for classmates to provide them with information and explanations and to provide answers to their questions.

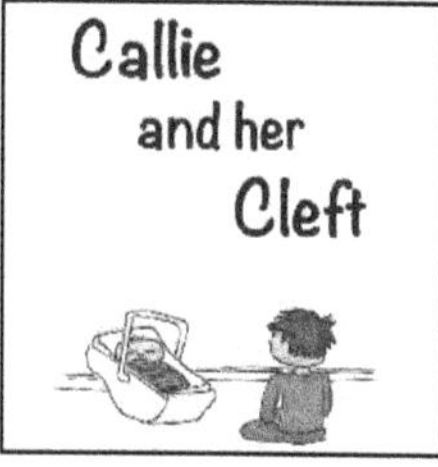

The booklet *'Callie and her Cleft'* can be downloaded for free from the website of the Cleft Lip and Palate Association (CLAPA), see https://www.clapa.com/product/callie-and-her-cleft/ . It was written to explain to brothers and sisters what it means when a new baby comes with a cleft lip or palate.

'The Broken Smile', written by Gulmakai Saleh and illustrated by Hira Shakir, is a beautiful picture book about a young girl who was born with a cleft lip. Then she learns that her smile is powerful enough to make other persons feel happy and better about themselves. The book was inspired by Gulmakai's granddaughter, who was born prematurely with a cleft lip, gum, and palate four years earlier.

We found a few **books for the youth**, featuring characters with CP.

Trent Reedy, who himself served as a soldier in Afghanistan, wrote *'Words in the Dust'*. The book is about the Afghan Zulaikha, who is born with protruding teeth and a prominent lip cleft. She is teased and mocked by the children in the neighborhood and sometimes even by her little brother. She hopes for peace now that the Taliban have been chased out so that she may be able to go back to school and, who knows, have surgery on her face. Then a number of things seem to fall into place. She is spotted by an American soldier who succeeds in convincing his superior to have her taken to a hospital for free surgery. She also meets a friend of her dead mother, who is willing to teach her to read. In addition, her

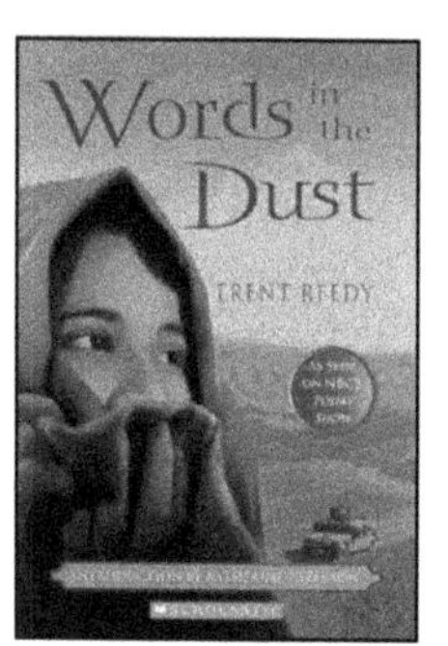

older sister is getting married. But beautiful dreams are sometimes smashed and that is what Zulaikha experiences. For children and young people from 10 to 11 years old.

'Before the Lark' is an award winning book, written by Irene Bennett Brown (2011). The story is set in 1888. Twelve-year-old Jocey, living in Kansas City, Missouri, who has a cleft lip, no longer goes to school. She believes that she will never have a friend, that others will always make fun of her, as they did at school before she quit. Since her mother died and her father became a drifter, Jocey has lived with her grandmother, a washerwoman. When she's not helping grandmother with laundry, she fills her lonely life with books and dreams. She prefers to be invisible. Mostly she dreams of Kansas and the farm her father abandoned there. On the farm, she could live in isolation—free from torment. Eventually she persuades her grandma to go with her to Kansas to life on the farm. Life on the farm is not, however, what she expected. Hard work was no surprise, but there are neighbours and traveling salesmen who cannot be avoided. Then there's grandmother, who seems determined to be sickly. Jocey wonders if she made a terrible mistake, until she discovers that any girl can have friends, if she will open herself to others. And she discovers that something can be done about her cleft lip too. For children 8 to 12 years old.

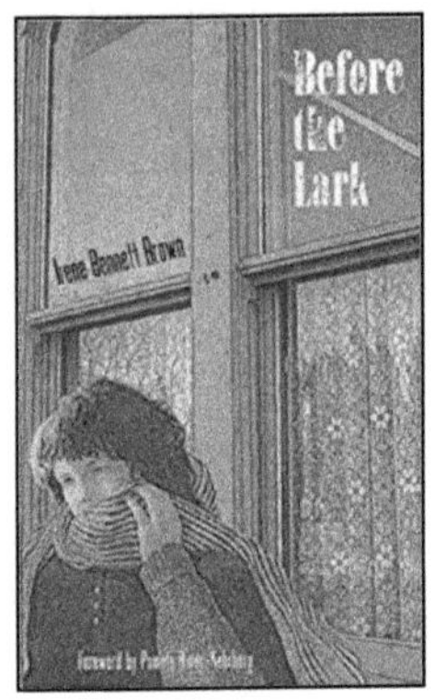

Chris Struyk-Bonn's *'Whisper'* is a book for children aged 12 to 16. Whisper is a 16-year-old girl with a cleft lip and palate. She lives with three other "outcasts" and their caretaker Nathanael in a community in the forest. When her mother, who visits her once a year, dies, she leaves her a violin. Nathanael teaches her how to play it. Then her father comes to take her back to the village, forcing her to run the household instead of her mother.

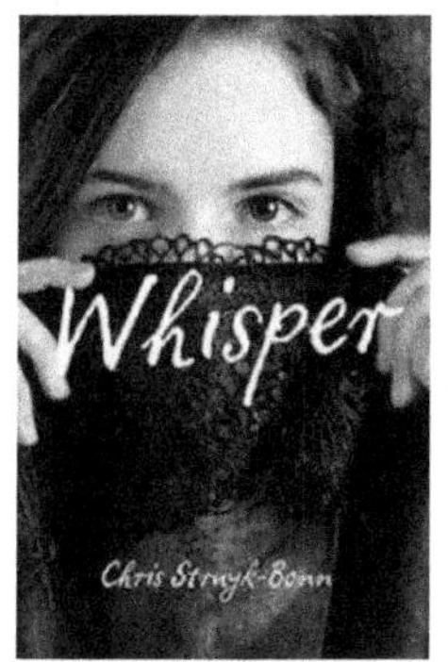

He makes her his house slave, who has to hide her face behind a black veil. However, she rebels against him and together with a number of companions she flees to the city, where they live together. In the meantime, her musical talent has also been discovered. Later on she has to make some tough decisions, both for herself and for her vulnerable friends.

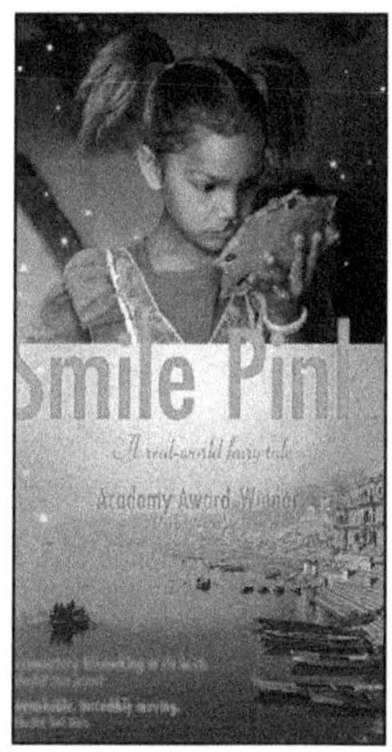

We also give two examples of **documentary films** about cleft lip and palate,. The first is the Oscar-winning film *'Smile Pinki'* from 2008, directed by Megan Mylan. This film focuses on a girl with a cleft lip in one of the poorest parts of India. A committed social worker makes every effort to get her to a hospital to repair the cleft. It also examines the traditions of the village where the girl lives and the popular belief that her cleft was caused by a solar eclipse. All in all, an uplifting story about how things turn out right after first being bad.

'Faces of Tomorrow' is a short (12 minutes) documentary film, directed by Meg Pinsonneault (2009). It sketches the work of Dr Brian Rubinstein, the Chief Pediatric Otolaryngology of Head and Neck Surgery, Facial Plastics and Reconstructive Surgery at Kaiser Permanente in Sacramento California and his team. In 2007, Dr Rubinstein founded 'Faces of Tomorrow', an non-profit organization that provides medical treatment to an underserved population of children, youth, and adults in developing countries, who might otherwise not receive the benefit of surgical treatments for their cleft lip or cleft. Faces of Tomorrow provides all their own medical supplies and raises

all the funds to be able to perform the operations for free. The organization does much more than repairing faces, they bring hope, happiness, and a new beginning to many families in need.

Voice disorders - laryngectomy

A voice disorder can be defined as a problem with pitch, volume, tone or other qualities of the voice. These problems usually occur when the vocal cords don't vibrate normally.

Laryngectomy is the surgical removal of part or all of the larynx, mostly due to laryngeal cancer.

On the internet a number of (auto)biographical stories of people with voice problems can be found. By way of illustration, we mention the story of the well-known actress and singer Julie Andrews (famous for her roles in the films 'Mary Poppins' and 'The sound of music'), who had to undergo surgery on her vocal cords in 1997 to free her from a benign lesion (vocal cord polyp or cyst?), but who had lost her singing voice after surgery. However, she was told that it was a minor, harmless procedure and that she would be able to sing again a few weeks later.

The book *'When do you talk normally again-how to deal with a voice disorder?'* (original title: Wanneer praat jij weer eens normaal-omgaan met een stemstoornis) tells the story of Dutch Marjolein Haze. She wrote it for people with a voice disorder and for (future) speech therapists. She describes the changes in life one undergoes when developing a voice disorder and how can be dealt with it. She also writes about the sometimes special and comical reactions of people when they hear a vulnerable voice.

In *'The voice gallery: Travels with a glass throat'*, Keath Fraser describes how he developed a rare voice disorder that almost made him voiceless. He was eventually diagnosed with spastic dysphonia, caused by incorrect control of the vocal cords by the brain.

At first he was told that his voice problems were psychological, but by applying botulinum toxin injections (botox) he regained

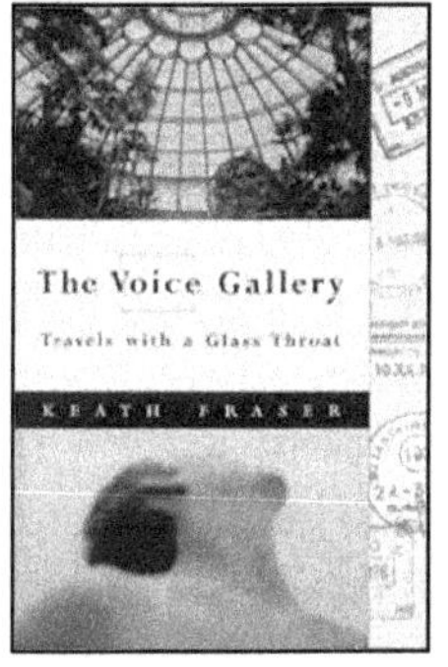

better control over his voice organ. All this spurred him to look for others who had also experienced such a mysterious drop in voice. He started his search on the Canadian west coast, but also traveled to New Zealand, South Africa, Great Britain, Ireland, the US, India and Sri Lanka. *'The Voice Gallery'* is an account of Fraser's international search for "lost voices". He had many conversations with individuals who had been through the same thing, among them some of the most astute minds and specialists. The book offers a good overview of the miracle, but also of the fragility of the human voice.

'Dumb, living without a voice' by Georgia Webber is partly autobiographic and partly a medical cautionary tale. The book

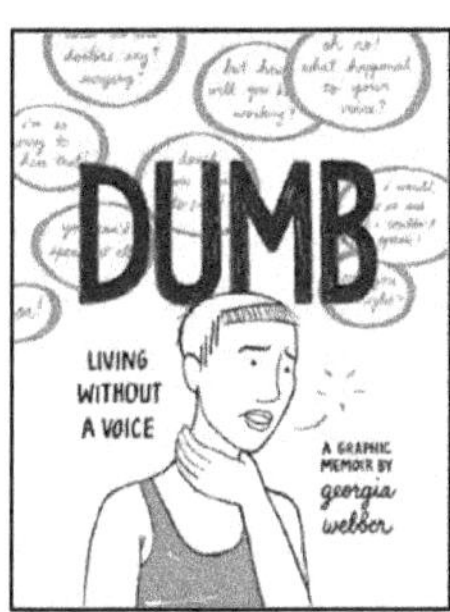

tells the story of how an young urban is trying to cope with the everyday challenges related to voicelessness. It is not very clear how she lost it, exactly, but in part it might be due to stress, to not taking take care of it properly or to abusing it. Everything changes for her, because she has to communicate through texting, through writing messages as she talks to other people. The author uses the comics medium to convey the practical hurdles she had to face as well as the fear and dread that accompanied her increasingly lonely journey to regain her life. Her raw cartooning style, occasionally devolving into chaotic scribbles, splotches of ink, and overlapping montages, perfectly captures her frustration and anxiety. But her ordeal ultimately becomes a hopeful story. Throughout, she learns to lean on the support of her close friends, finds self-expression in creating comics, and comes to understand and appreciate how deeply her voice and identity are intertwined.

To build a bridge to laryngectomy, we first mention *'When David Lost His Voice'* by the Belgian Judith Vanistendael. This beautiful graphic novel tells the story of the bookseller David, who has been told that he has developed laryngeal cancer, and how he himself and his various family members deal with it. Vanistendael indicates that the book is not autobiographical, but that she has been confronted with cancer a number of times in recent years and that she drew on those experiences. The story was actually already in her head when she started it. It starts at the intersection between life and death: Miriam gives birth to her first child and soon after she learns that her father has cancer. Tamar, David's youngest daughter, explores what death means and how to keep a soul alive. Paula can't accept her husband's abandonment. David himself especially wants to make one more beautiful journey.

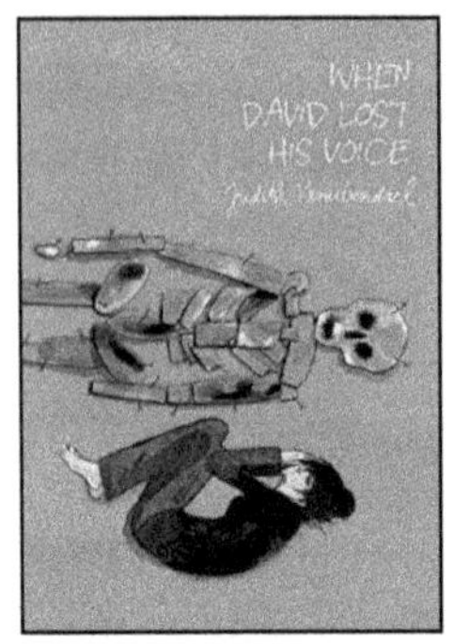

'Speechless - My Laryngectomy Story' is written by Jo Jenner. During what should have been a routine thyroidectomy the surgeon spots a shadow on the CT scan. What follows are tests, operations, scar tissue, complications and more operations.Jo had to breathe through a tracheostomy tube for six months, was fed through a tube for twelve months and was unable to speak for twelve weeks. This is her story of how she made it through a partial laryngectomy with some of the best care the NHS had to offer.

'A few restless cells' (original Dutch title: *'Een paar rusteloze cellen'*) is an autobiographical story by Willem Harting about the diagnosis of pulmonary emphysema, the treatment of and

living with a precancerous stage of laryngeal cancer. It is an easily readable book that also provides insight in what may still play a role after cancer treatment.

Willem Melchior describes in *'The time is up'* (original Dutch title *'De tijd is op'*) how he was told to have laryngeal cancer in the summer of 2012. He is subject to a program of examinations, counseling and treatment and has to quit smoking. This means that he - an enthusiastic smoker - also has to reinvent his daily life as a writer. From day to day he registers what happens to him, examining himself mercilessly: fear, fatalism and resignation compete to assert themselves.

The sequel to this book is called *'All That Was'* (Dutch title: *'Alles wat was'*). Herein Melchior describes his further disease process. His larynx will be removed in 2014. The book is about the change he had to make spiritually, mentally and finally emotionally to come to accept his fate in the months leading up to the operation. Suicide becomes a serious option, faith is gaining in significance. What do you have to do in order to live? How do you survive when death threatens? Can a man bear to be forgotten? And what about his mother? In this book Melchior shows us man in his utmost nakedness, loneliness and vulnerability.

We did also find two autobiographical French books on laryngectomy.

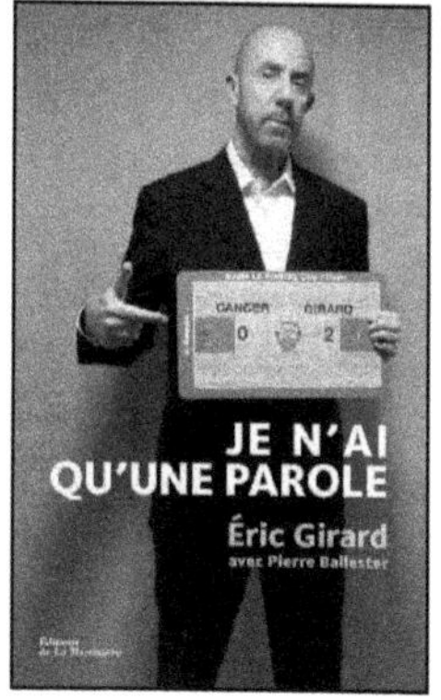

'Je n'ai qu'une parole' (I just have one word) was written by the Frenchman Eric Girard, a former famous basketball player and coach. He underwent a partial laryngectomy in 2011, followed by a total laryngectomy a year later. For this great sportsman of course his laryngeal cancer could mean the end of the world or in any case of his world. Despite his illness he

fights back and nowadays he's the coach of the 'Le Portel'-team, with which he realizes miracles.

The life story of Nadine Ilopsis, written down by Estelle Loiseau, is titled '*Et si j'en parlais…*' (And what if I talked about it…). At 32, Nadine underwent a partial laryngectomy, at 48, her cancer had recurred and she had to undergo total laryngectomy. She had to learn everything again: to talk, to eat, to drink, in a word, to live.

'*Can You Hear My Voice?*' is a **documentary film** about the transition from life with a voice box to one without. This film is told through the personal accounts of members of the 'Shout at Cancer Choir' in London, made up of individuals who have undergone laryngectomy. Throughout the film, the choir members share their personal experiences of life after surgery and overcoming the obstacles of living as a laryngectomee as they prepare for and perform a special concert.

In the **horror-film** '*Us*' by Jordan Peele from 2019, the actress Lupita Nyong'o is playing a character, suffering from spasmodic dysphonia, a condition mentioned earlier when we described Keath Fraser's book. Nyong'o later had to endure a lot of criticism from the National Spasmodic Dysphonia Association, because she would have demonized the condition. The actress later apologized, stating it was not at all her intention to offend people suffering from this kind of dysphonia.

Childhood speech and language disorders

A developmental language disorder (DLD) occurs in children whose language difficulties are not associated with a known biomedical condition, such as brain injury, cerebral palsy, sensorineural hearing loss, ASD or intellectual disability.

Some books are intended in the first place for parents and supervisors of children with speech and language disorders. After all, despite growing awareness about DLD, there are not so many books available to help parents and children understand and cope with this condition.

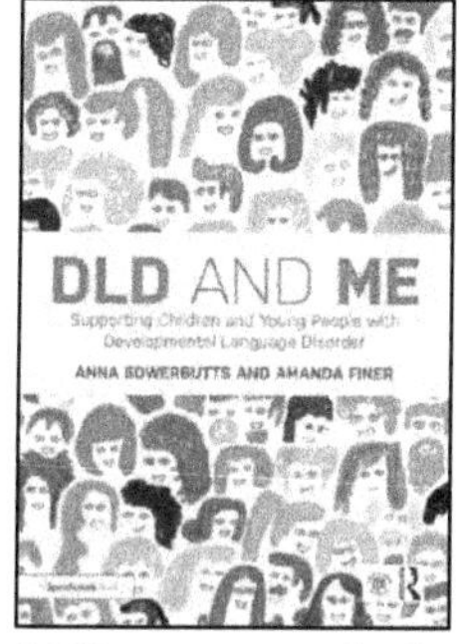

The book *'DLD and Me: Supporting Children and Young People with Developmental Language Disorder'*, written by Anna Sowerbutts and Amanda Finer, aims to address this need. It provides a source of information for young and slightly older children, parents and families. It examines the strengths of people with TOS, what makes them different and how they themselves can improve their communication in everyday life.

The fifth edition (2017) of *'It Takes Two to Talk: A Practical Guide For Parents of Children With Language Delays'* by Elaine Weitzman, gives parents a tool to stimulate their child's language in a natural way, so that language intervention becomes a natural, ongoing part of everyday life with their child. The book is intended for parents and caregivers of young children who need extra help in stimulating their speech and language. It teaches them methods and skills to improve communicative interaction with their child. The premise is that parents are constantly present in their young children's lives, much more often than the experts, and are thus best placed to optimize their child's language skills in all kinds of everyday situations.

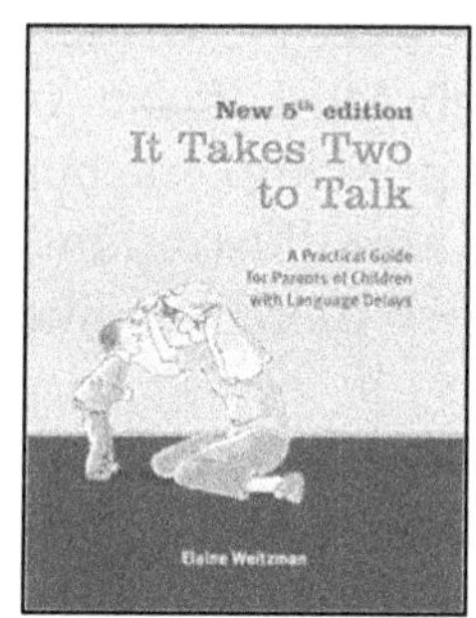

In the first chapter of this latest edition new checklists and goal charts make it easier for parents and professionals to identify the child's stage of communication and to choose the most appropriate interaction and communication goals. With a heightened focus on helping children initiate, take turns in enjoyable, extended interactions and increase their expressive language skills, this guidebook shows parents how responsive interaction strategies can be used, that increase children's language skills. Written in simple language and beautifully illustrated by Pat Cupples, this book is the ideal guide to show parents how to integrate Hanen's *'It Takes Two to Talk'*-strategies into everyday routines like mealtime, bath time, playtime and reading books with children.

Although Childhood Apraxia of Speech (CAS) is a rather exceptional condition, several books relate to this condition. As defined by the American Speech-Language-Hearing Association (ASHA) CAS is a neurological childhood (pediatric) speech sound disorder in which the precision and consistency of movements underlying speech are impaired in the absence of neuromuscular deficits.

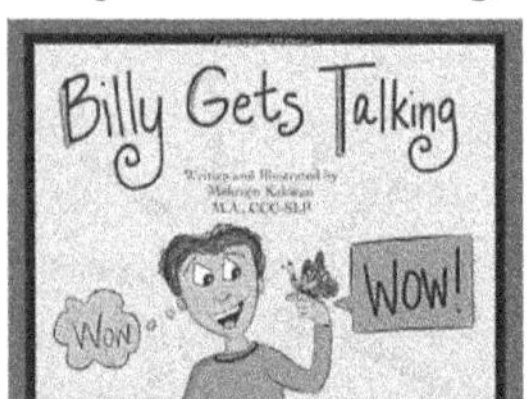

'Billy Gets Talking: A Preschooler's Journey Overcoming Childhood Apraxia of Speech' , written and illustrated by Mehreen Kakwan, is a book suitable for preschoolers but also elementary with nice illustrations. It describes what speech therapy is like for a child with CAS. It is also very illuminating for parents and for therapists. For the latter explaining to parents and caregivers what CAS is can sometimes be really difficult. This book can allow parents to better understand the difficult journey of a child who wants to communicate, but has to struggle very hard to do so. It's a book parents can read with their children, but it's also a nice book to share with other family members.

It can be coupled with *'Let's Get Talking. A Speech-Language Therapy Companion for a Child's First Functional Words'*, also written by Mehreen Kakwan. It is presented as a speech-language therapy companion guide for parents of children, who are diagnosed with an expressive language delay or disorder, or with childhood apraxia of speech (CAS). Carry-over of skills from therapy to the home environment increases the rate of success as your child is learning to produce their first words. The verbal and tactile cues, as well as visual signs and prompts described can be used to help children meet their next achievable step in functional communication, and to reduce communicative frustration. The author presents a wealth of information on speech and language development and on specific activities to be used with children to help them with their first sounds, syllables and words.

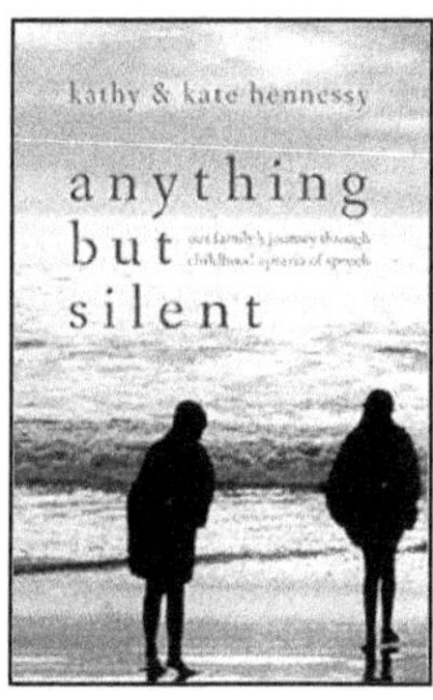

Most parents dream that their children will accomplish many great things, but they do not dream that their children will struggle for years just to learn to say what is in their hearts and minds. Kathy Hennessy, the author of *'Anything but Silent: Our Family's Journey Through Childhood Apraxia of Speech'* faced this challenge when not one but both of her children were diagnosed with childhood apraxia of speech. What does a child feel like when no one in the world understands what she is trying to say? Imagine the frustration when even your mom doesn't get it. In this straightforward and emotional story, Kathy tells of the mountains they climbed just for her children to have a chance at speech and of the battles she waged with insurance companies, paediatricians, school systems, and family members. A heartbreaking account.

A wacky speech teacher starts swallowing everything she needs to do speech/language therapy in her school! What could possibly happen? *'There Was a Speech Teacher Who Swallowed Some Dice'* by Patricia Mervine is a delightfully silly way to introduce students to many of the materials used in speech therapy, and ends with a Speech Room Scavenger Hunt. This story is both educational (explaining a speech teachers role and the items they use) and a cool ice breaker for children who may be attending speech class.

Denise Voccola wrote *'Tessa's Tangled Tongue'*. Tessa is a girl, who's tongue gets tangled sometimes. Because of that her words don't always come out exactly as they should.

But when that happens, she doesn't get mad or frustrated. She thinks it's funny and so will readers! Moms and children with speech delays will be encouraged by Tessa's unique way of dealing with the frustration of not always being understood. This book would be great for all children, but especially for those with a speech delay or any other "difference" or disability. It shows clearly that not every child communicates in spoken words, but this hardly means they have nothing to say.

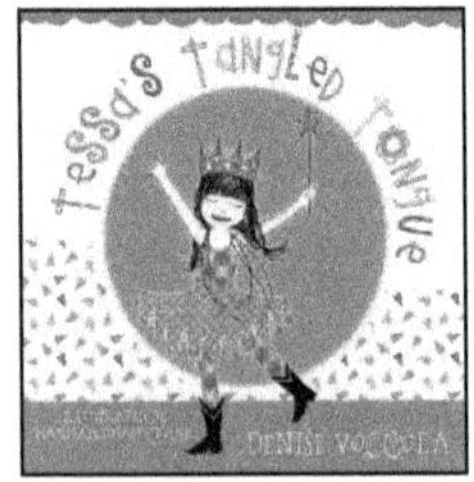

'Beyond Words: : A Child's Journey Through Apraxia', written by Dana Hall, is presented as a valuable social-emotional teaching tool, that will compliment any home library, school, speech language program, or classroom. Through beautiful illustrations and thoughtful text, it draws a picture of the inner world of children that have differences that others can't see and thus increases our understanding of CAS. A lot of children with speech/language problems such as Apraxia of Speech often feel isolated and alone. Beyond Words can help to create an understanding of what life with a communication disorder feels like not only for the child concerned but also for the child's peers.

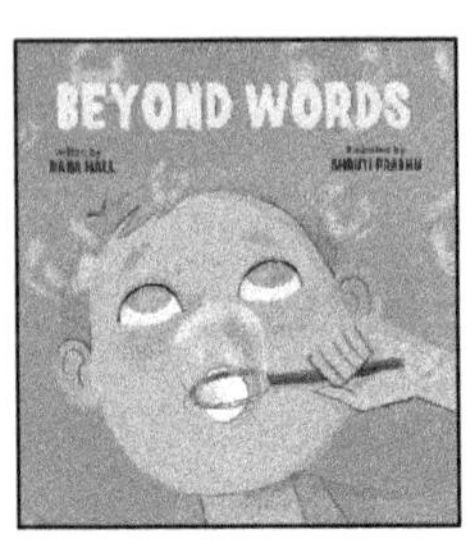

'The Mouth With a Mind of Its Own' by Patricia Mervine (speech therapist) and Nayan Soni follows the little boy Michael, who also shows a speech apraxia.

His mouth doesn't want to cooperate with what his brain wants to say. The booklet discusses the problems he

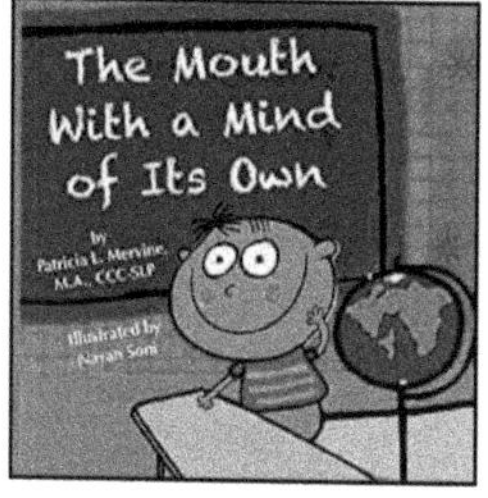

experiences at school and during speech therapy, as well as the frustration associated with having a serious speech disorder. This book can give children, who experience the same problem, a companion who has also been through it all. For children from 4 to 8 years old.

'Hi, my name is Milly' by Heather Zeissler is about CAS as well. Older sister Milly has a special bond with her little brother Malcolm, who shows apraxia of speech. Through her story we learn how on the one hand the whole family is influenced by little brother's limited verbal skills, but on the other hand his development is positively stimulated thanks to the help and support of the family. This booklet not only brings awareness to the condition, but also shows that children with apraxia can be sensible, something that is sometimes masked by their verbal limitations.

Some books relate to more general speech problems than CAS.

'Something to Say about My Speech' by Eden Molineux is about the girl Macey. She loves adventure and taking charge. But she

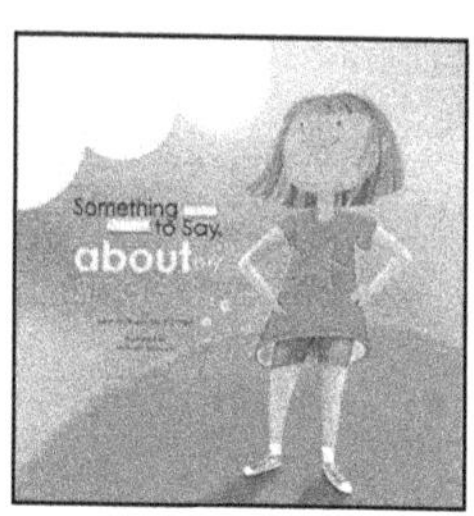

also has a speech problem. In this book she shares her experiences about her speech while at the same time enjoying being a child just like her friends. The booklets from the *'Something to Say'* series promote self-advocacy, better understanding of differences in speech and language, and engage in a conversation about diversity. Written by a speech therapist, each book presents a character with a communication problem. The strengths and interests of the children are highlighted and the reader gains insight into how he/she can promote communication. In this series also the booklet

'Something to say about my stuttering' was published, written by the same author.

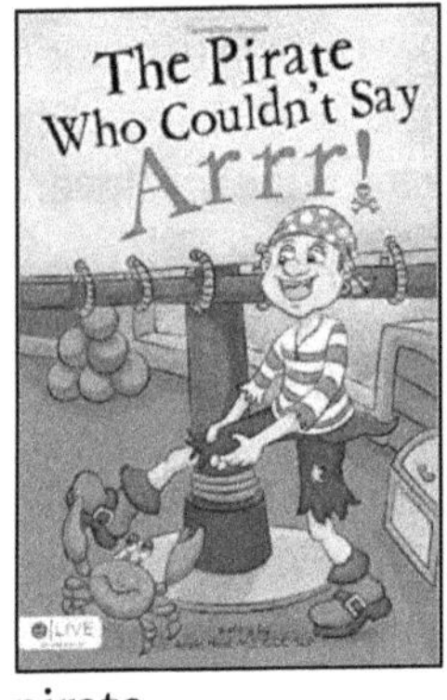

Two booklets deal with articulation problems. In *'The Pirate Who Couldn't Say Arrr!'* by speech therapist Angie Neal, the pirate Red Legs cannot pronounce the pirate battle cry "Arrr", which is of course a disadvantage in his profession. In this booklet, we follow his adventures across the seas and the oceans and see how he eventually manages to utter the cry and how everyone can learn to speak like a pirate.

Helen Lester's *'Hooway for Wodney Wat'* is about Rodney Rat, who cannot pronounce the speech sound "R" and is therefore teased by the other rodents in the class. When Camilla Capybara ends up in Rodney's class and she says that she's bigger, nastier and smarter than everyone else, everyone is scared, until the moment our hero Wodney beats her without wanting to in a game. To his own great surprise, he saves himself and the entire class, with or without "R".

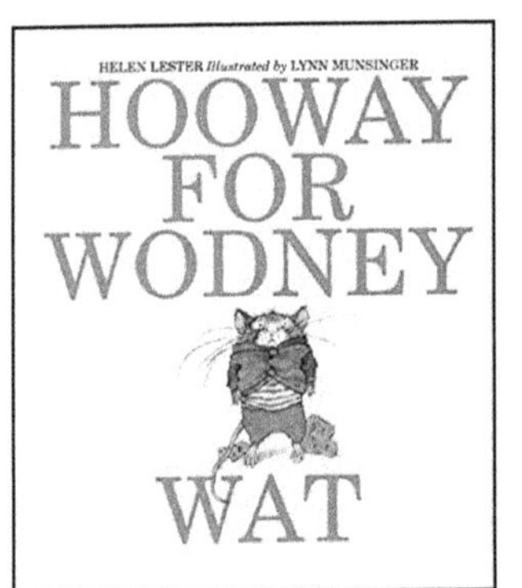

The following two somewhat similar booklets are meant both for children with a speech problem and their parents. *'Aiden Goes to Speech'* was written by Lisa Mortensen and illustrated by Maryna Salagub.

It is the ideal booklet for parents whose children are experiencing speech difficulties. It is a fascinating story about a little boy who, as a result of his speech difficulties, suffers from feelings of confusion, frustration and even loneliness. He eventually ends up in a nice speech class, where he flourishes. Very suitable for children from the age of 4, but also for parents, educators and speech therapists to achieve understanding, empathy and acceptance.

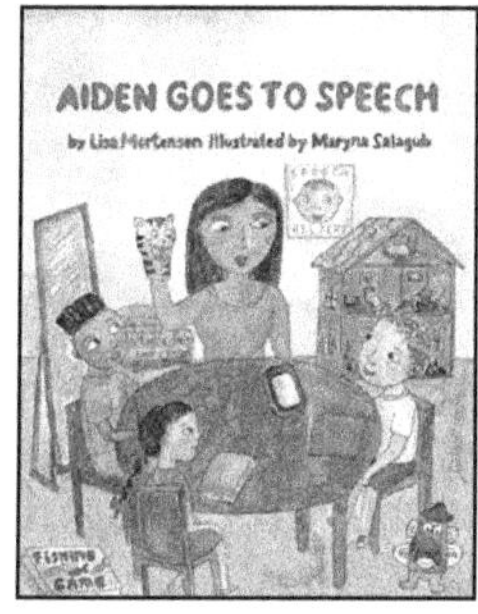

In *'Sammy goes to speech'* by Marisa Siegel, Sammy wants to communicate, but he doesn't succeed. Sammy and his family look for help in search of his speech. After searching everywhere they end up with a speech therapist. Sammy is learning to develop his speech and language together with his pet, Mr. Monster, and with his Mommy.

As far as **audiovisual media** are concerned, we found some animated films featuring characters with speech difficulties. For example, in the Looney Tunes series *'Duck Season - Wabbit Season'*, both the hunter and the duck show clear problems with the pronunciation of the "r" and the "l" sound. The figure *'Tweety'*, also from the Looney Tunes series, has problems with the pronunciation of the "s"-sound. Disney's *'Robin Hood'* (1973) also features some animal figures with pronunciation problems.

In the gangster comedy *'Snatch'* (2000) directed by Guy Ritchie, Brad Pitt plays a gypsy who talks completely unintelligible. The film is set in London and revolves around a huge stolen diamond as well as troubles in the local illegal boxing circuit.

We find a completely different, but very fascinating theme in the French film *'L' Enfant Sauvage'* (The Wild Child of Aveyron) made by François Truffaut in 1970. It tells the story of the wild boy Victor and is based on true facts. The boy was found in the wilderness in the late eighteenth century, when he was about twelve years old. He was unable to walk upright, speak, and of course didn't read or write. He fed on carrots, nuts and potatoes. The news of his discovery spreads quickly and comes to the attention of the general public. He is transferred to an institution for deaf-mute children near Paris, where he becomes an attraction for the well-to-do Parisians for a while. However, people quickly lose their interest in the 'wild child' and the doctors become convinced that he cannot be educated. They therefore want to transfer him to a specialized institution, where he cannot harm anyone. Ultimately, an interested doctor, Dr. Jean Itard, asks permission to make an attempt to raise the child. Although he was a medical doctor, Itard is considered by many to be one of the first historical figures in the field of speech and language pathology. He tried, not with undivided success, to apply a number of scientific principles from phonetics and linguistics to Victor's education. Itard himself described his findings regarding this feral boy in the work *'De l'education d'un homme sauvage ou des premiers développements physiques et moraux du jeune sauvage de l'Aveyron'* (On the education of a savage man or on the first physical and moral developments of the young savage of Aveyron) (1801). The complete film (with English subtitles) can be found on the vimeo-channel[16]. Although a little outdated it is still worth watching.

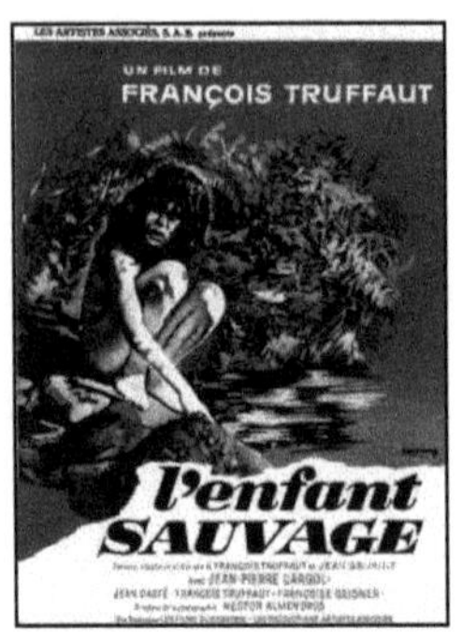

[16] See https://vimeo.com/215596192

In the book *'Wild Child'* T.C. Boyle also tells the story of Victor. A very detailed, scientifically based description of this case can be found in *'The Wild Boy of Aveyron'* by Harlan Lane (1976).

References chapter 7

Bastidas, N, Scabuso, N. (2019). *Beth and her Cleft.* Independently published, s.l.

Bennett Brown, I. (2011). *Before the Lark.* Texas Tech University Press, Lubbock.

Boyle, T.C., (2010). *Wild Child and Other Stories.* Viking books, New York.

Fraser, K. (2002). *The voice gallery: Travels with a glass throat.* Thomas Allen publishers, Markham.

Gaynor, K. (2007). *First place.* Special Stories Publishing, Dublin.

Girard, E. 2016). *Je n'ai qu'une parole.* La Martinière, Paris.

Gore, B. (2011). *Zoe, a cool cleft kid.* Beth Gore, s.l.

Graham, J. (2006). *A Special Smile.* Trafford Publishing, Bloomington.

Gulmakai, S., Shakir, H. (2020). *The Broken Smile.* Independently published, s.l.

Hall, D. (2020). *Beyond Words: A Child's Journey Through Apraxia.* Tecassia Publishing, London.

Harting, W. (2010). *Een paar onrustige cellen.* Uitgeverij Boekscout, Utrecht.

Haze, M. (2018). *Wanneer praat jij nou weer eens normaal? - Omgaan met een stemstoornis.* Uitgeverij Boekscout, Utrecht. .

Hennessy, K. (2019*). Anything but Silent: Our Family's Journey Through Childhood Apraxia of Speech.* Word Association Publishers

Ilopsis, N. (2020). *Et si j'en parlais.* Published by Estelle Loiseau, Pontacq.

Itard, J.M.G (1801). *'De l'education d'un homme sauvage ou des premiers développements physiques et moraux du jeune sauvage de l'Aveyron*. Editions Gouyon, Paris.

Jenner, J. (2016). *Speechless - My Laryngectomy Story*. Kindle Edition.

Johnston-Burnham, M. (2013). *Cleft Talk for Kids*. CreateSpace Independent Publishing Platform, Scotts Valley.

Kummer, A. (2008). *Cleft palate and craniofacial anomalies*. Delmar Cengage Learning, Clifton Park.

Lane, H. (1976). *The Wild Boy of Aveyron*. Bantam books, New York.

Lester, H. (1999). *Hooway for Wodney Wat*. Houghton Mifflin Harcourt, New York.

Lipman, B. *'My Puzzling Smile'*, s.n., s.l.

Kakwan, M. (2018). *Billy Gets Talking: : A Preschooler's Journey Overcoming Childhood Apraxia of Speech*. Independently published, s.l.

Kakwan, M. (2019). *Let's Get Talking: A Speech-Language Therapy Companion for a Child's First Functional Words*. Independently published, s.l.

Melchior, W. (2014). *De tijd is op*. Atlas Contact, Amsterdam.

Melchior W. (2018). *Alles wat was*. Atlas Contact, Amsterdam.

Mervine, P. Soni, N. (2014). *The Mouth With a Mind of Its' Own*. Speaking of Speech.com., Inc., New York

Mervine, P. (2014). *There Was a Speech Teacher Who Swallowed Some Dice*. CreateSpace Independent Publishing Platform, Scotts Valley.

Molineux, E. (2017). *Something to Say about My Speech*. Something to Say-series, London.

Mortensen, L. (2018). *Aiden Goes to Speech*. CreateSpace Independent Publishing Platform, Scotts Valley. .

Neal, A. (2011). *The Pirate Who Couldn't Say Arrr!*. Tate Publishing, London.

Reedy, T. (2013). *Words in the dust*. Scholastic USA.

Saman, M., Gross, J., Ovchinsky, A.., Wood-Smith, D. (2012). Cleft Lip and Palate in the Arts: A Critical Reflection. *Cleft Palate–Craniofacial Journal*, 49 (2); 129-136.

Siegel, M. (2018). *Sammy Goes to Speech.* CreateSpace Independent Publishing Platform, Scotts Valley.
Simon, P.A. (2017). *Smile with Simon*. Published by Patricia Ann Simon, s.l.
Sowerbutts, A., Finer, A. (2019). *DLD and Me: Supporting Children and Young People with Developmental Language Disorder*. Routledge, London.
Struyk-Bonn, C. (2014). *Whisper*. Orca books, Custer.
Trivelpiece, R.M., West, S., Rhodes, J. Nunez, B. (2017). *Jack's New Smile: Having a baby with cleft lip and palate.* CreateSpace Independent Publishing Platform, Scotts Valley.
Vanistendael, J. (2013). *When David lost his Voice.* SelfMadeHero, London.
Vermeylen-Nuyts, M. (2008). *Katie's dream.* BAI-NV, Kontich.
Voccola, D. (2017*). Tessa's tangled tongue*. CreateSpace Independent Publishing Platform, Scotts Valley.
Weitzman, E. (2017, 5th ed.). *It Takes Two to Talk: A Practical Guide For Parents of Children With Language Delays. Published by The Hanen Centre.* Toronto.
Zeissler, H. (2013). *Hi, my name is Milly*. Theacq, s.l.

General Conclusion

As mentioned earlier, Baskin and Harris (1984) pointed out that purely informational books typically have only a moderate influence in establishing or changing attitudes. In contrast, fiction stories and films allow readers and viewers to identify with particular characters and to share their emotions, imitate their behavior, and share or, on the contrary, reject their perceptions and judgments.

Fictional stories can also help people to see how they can or cannot respond to persons with certain disabilities or abnormalities. Indeed, there are arguments to claim that fiction stories not only have the potential to influence the reader's thoughts, emotions, and attitudes toward particular problems, but can also provide new and fresh ideas and insights about how to respond or not to respond and how can be dealt with problems. For the individuals themselves who exhibit speech, language, hearing or other communication difficulties, books and/or films can be a resource to help them understand that others have experienced and often overcome similar problems as theirs, have somehow learned to cope with it or have learned to live with it. In this way, books can also be very useful tools in so-called bibliotherapy. This refers to the process of reading, reflecting upon, and discussing literature, often first person illness or disability narratives, to promote cognitive shifts in the way clients and clinicians conceptualize the experience of disability. As Gerlach and Subramanian (2016) showed, bibliotherapy can be used as an effective tool in therapy of PWS and also in clinical education.

Susan Sontag stated in her book *'Illness as a metaphor'* (1978, quoted in Eagle, 2014) that metaphorical associations and resulting moral judgments are often projected onto a variety of illnesses and disorders. Since speech, language and hearing disorders are not terminal disorders and, moreover, in many cases entail few visible limitations, they occupy only a marginal position in the fields of medical sciences and in disability studies. Nevertheless speech, language and hearing impairments do often not escape from pejorative judgments.

Unfortunately many books and films do indeed stigmatize people with speech, language or hearing problems. Negative stereotyping is very common. Traits such as nervousness and frailty are often discussed, but even sexual inexperience or even impotence are sometimes, completely incorrectly, listed as being typical of persons with speech disorders. Sudden outbursts of aggression or violence to compensate for their verbal inability are also described in some books or shown in certain films. Think back to the character Billy Budd, the boxer Rubin "Hurricane" Carter or the girl Merry in Philip Roth's *'American Pastoral'*. Often people with speech, language or hearing problems are also seen as stupid, ridiculous or pitiful. The latter trend is particularly regrettable in people who stutter. We see a prototypical example of this in the film *'A fish called Wanda'*.

However, when reading excerpts from books or watching scenes from films, we noticed how strong and resilient some people with communication problems turn out to be. During our search we found a lot of books and films drawing a picture of very strong and courageous individuals, who have often found a way to cope with and adapt to their impairments. Especially in (auto) biographies and documentary films it is sometimes clear that many of them have adapted admirably to their limitations and try to "make the best of it", even with their limited or reduced verbal and communicative capabilities. This is the case, among others, in people who became aphasic after a heavy brain hemorrhage or in persons who ended up in a locked-in condition after a brain stem injury. A number of their stories about their illness, sometimes achieved with great difficulty, are even downright optimistic in tone and hopeful for fellow sufferers. Many deaf or hard of hearing people embrace ‘Deaf Culture’ in all its aspects and don’t even consider themselves as disabled, as they believe -quite rightly- that they are completely equivalent to hearing persons.

If we look at children's and young adult books, featuring characters with speech, language and hearing difficulties, it struck us that the stories are often very optimistic. They often emphasize the strengths of the children concerned. For example, a child with a stuttering problem enters a new class, is first teased or laughed at, but then manifests himself as a terrific football player, is appreciated as a result, gains self-confidence and for that reason starts to speak more fluently. In a number of cases we wonder whether things aren’t presented a bit too rosy from time to time. Of course it’s beyond doubt that these children's and young adult books can be used to increase the understanding of some of these problems, heighten their acceptance and provide role models to the children concerned. Some of them are explicitly intended for that goal.

We fully realize that we have told only part of the story in this book and that it is absolutely incomplete in some aspects. As mentioned in the introduction, we have chosen not to include communication problems caused by other underlying conditions, such as autism or dementia. After all, this would have taken us very far, because a great deal has been published about these disorders. Who knows, this could maybe provide with material for a next book.

Nevertheless, we hope to have broadened the horizon somewhat with this publication. After all, there are many scientific texts in the form of articles and handbooks on the described problems, but as far as we know little has been published until now about speech, language and hearing problems in the so-called "popular" media. The work is of course not finished yet. Therefore it would be our pleasure to receive feedback and to get any additions from readers. Anyone who knows about (children's) books, films or other media in which people with speech, language and/or hearing problems appear and who are not mentioned by us, may always report this to us (manders.eric@scarlet.be).

Appendix: selected list of websites consulted

https://www.goodreads.com/list/show/6168.Selective_Mutism

https://www.verdermethersenletsel.nl/thema-s/boeken-over-niet-aangeboren-hersenletsel

https://www.amazon.com/Literature-Speech-Disorders-Disability-Interdisciplinary/dp/0415823048

https://iris.peabody.vanderbilt.edu/resources/films/

http://guides.library.illinois.edu/c.php?g=613892&p=4265885

https://www.bloomsbury.com/us/dysfluencies-9781623564629/

https://www.goodreads.com/book/show/14481464-life-after-stroke

https://www.goodreads.com/shelf/show/aphasia

https://www.patientervaringsverhalen.nl/?pagina=Aandoeningen

https://www.goodreads.com/list/show/37854.Fiction_Books_on_Stuttering

https://thelearningcorp.com/brainwire/the-curated-book-list-on-brain-injury-and-dementia-for-speech-language-pathologists/

https://www.goodreads.com/list/show/22561.Books_for_Speech_Language_Pathologists

https://en.wikipedia.org/wiki/My_Left_Foot_(book)

https://www.goodreads.com/list/show/61680.Books_about_H
earing_Loss

https://www.jeugdbibliotheek.nl/catalogus.catalogus.2.html?
d=dcterms%3Asubject%7CStotteren

http://www.aphasianow.org/Aphasia_Recovery/Aphasia_and
_Stroke_books/Aphasia_Related_Books/

https://books.google.be/books?id=LBBmDwAAQBAJ&pg=PT
20&lpg=PT20&dq=monsieur+noirtier+de+villefort+locked+in
&source=bl&ots=Lsj3O8ehMk&sig=ACfU3U3PggGr64agUYH8
7fFSHzUwQGxhUA&hl=nl&sa=X&ved=2ahUKEwi6oufwg4jnA
hWI6qQKHS8aCXoQ6AEwAXoECAwQAQ#v=onepage&q=m
onsieur%20noirtier%20de%20villefort%20locked%20in&f=fal
se

https://en.wikipedia.org/wiki/Stuttering_in_popular_culture

https://stutter.ca/articles/book-reviews/372-fictions-of-
stuttering-stories-of-dysfluency.html

https://seattle.bibliocommons.com/list/share/686344577/1193
275127

https://www.stutteringhelp.org/cuban-author-frequently-
wrote-about-stuttering

https://desingel.be/nl/programma/theater/nancy-gabor-
joseph-chaikin-texts-for-nothing

https://www.euppublishing.com/doi/pdfplus/10.3366/E03095
20709000090

https://www.scribd.com/document/47946589/1969-Samuel-
Beckett-Eh-Joe

https://www.goodreads.com/list/show/16469.Deaf_Mute_Spe
echless_Romance_Heroes_and_Heroines?fbclid=IwAR2gLTN
GbxbUTMo4glkdDpSMt4zFcRlK_r2PNkoiBYsb6LnnnCsdF2jf
XzE

http://www.bidocnet.be/doofvlaanderen/index.html?q=rubriek

https://en.wikipedia.org/wiki/List_of_films_featuring_the_deaf_and_hard_of_hearing

https://en.wikipedia.org/wiki/Stuttering_in_popular_culture#Literature

http://www.bidocnet.be/doofvlaanderen/index.html

https://www.mnsu.edu/comdis/kuster/media/songs.html

https://www.prospectmagazine.co.uk/magazine/david-mitchell-stammering-kings-speech

www.ingramcontent.com/pod-product-compliance
Ingram Content Group UK Ltd.
Pitfield, Milton Keynes, MK11 3LW, UK
UKHW021910190726
13853UKWH00002B/602

9 798536 720585